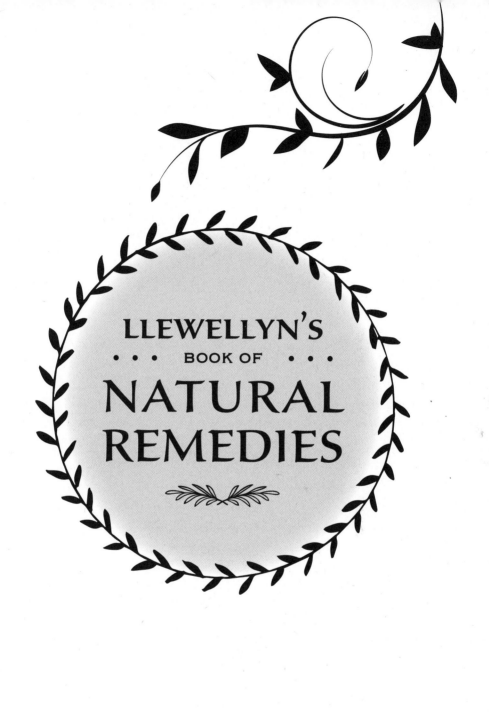

# LLEWELLYN'S
## • • • BOOK OF • • •
# NATURAL REMEDIES

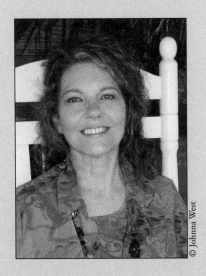
© Johnna West

## ABOUT THE AUTHOR

Vannoy Gentles Fite is the author of *Essential Oils for Healing* and currently lives in Saltillo, Texas. She is a certified Ayurvedic lifestyle coach, a certified herbalist, a licensed yoga instructor, and a certified aromatherapist. She believes wholeheartedly in natural healing methods, yoga, Ayurveda, and living mindfully and sustainably. She lives her life as spiritually as her path allows and is forever growing as a soul. Fite continues to grow her own vegetable garden and herbs, instructs and practices yoga, raises chickens, ducks, and fish, studies Ayurveda, and is a part of a beautiful family.

EM: vannoylou@gmail.com
FB: Vannoy Gentles Fite, Author
IG: @vannoylou
Amazon: www.amazon.com/author/vannoyfite
Goodreads: www.goodreads.com/goodreadscomauthor/vannoyfite

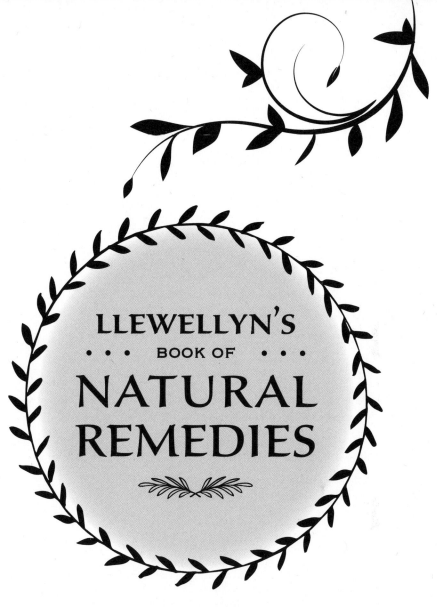

# LLEWELLYN'S
## • • • BOOK OF • • •
# NATURAL REMEDIES

OVER 400
AYURVEDIC, HERBAL,
ESSENTIAL OIL,
AND HOME REMEDIES FOR
EVERYDAY AILMENTS

## VANNOY GENTLES FITE

LLEWELLYN PUBLICATIONS
woodbury, minnesota

FIRST EDITION
Fifth Printing, 2023

Book design by Rebecca Zins
Cover design by Shira Atakpu

Llewellyn Publications is a registered trademark of Llewellyn Worldwide Ltd.

**Library of Congress Cataloging-in-Publication Data**
Names: Fite, Vannoy Gentles, author.
Title: Llewellyn's book of natural remedies : over 400 ayurvedic, herbal, essential oil, and home remedies for everyday ailments / Vannoy Gentles Fite.
Description: First edition. | Woodbury, Minnesota : Llewellyn Publications, [2020] | Includes bibliographical references. | Summary: "This book contains more than 400 remedies using everyday ingredients for 101 different ailments, with each ailment supported by four remedies, one from each category of essential oils, herbs, Ayurveda, and home remedies"—Provided by publisher.
Identifiers: LCCN 2020000923 (print) | LCCN 2020000924 (ebook) | ISBN 9780738762913 (paperback) | ISBN 9780738763125 (ebook)
Subjects: LCSH: Naturopathy. | Alternative medicine.
Classification: LCC RZ440 .F55 2020  (print) | LCC RZ440  (ebook) | DDC 615.5/35—dc23
LC record available at https://lccn.loc.gov/2020000923
LC ebook record available at https://lccn.loc.gov/2020000924

Llewellyn Worldwide Ltd. does not participate in, endorse, or have any authority or responsibility concerning private business transactions between our authors and the public.

All mail addressed to the author is forwarded, but the publisher cannot, unless specifically instructed by the author, give out an address or phone number.

Any internet references contained in this work are current at publication time, but the publisher cannot guarantee that a specific location will continue to be maintained. Please refer to the publisher's website for links to authors' websites and other sources.

Llewellyn Publications
A Division of Llewellyn Worldwide Ltd.
2143 Wooddale Drive
Woodbury, MN 55125-2989
www.llewellyn.com

Printed in the United States of America

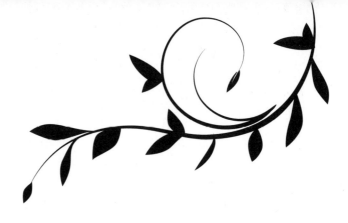

## SPECIAL DEDICATION

For my daughters, the best women I know,
Lin Reynolds and Colleen Hoover. There is no one
else I would have chosen to take this ride with.

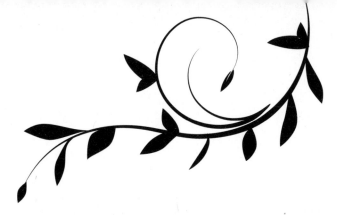

# CONTENTS

••••

# CONTENTS

# CONTENTS

• • • •

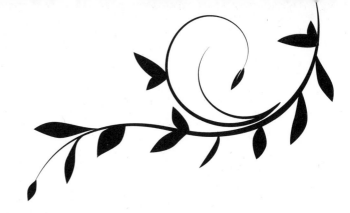

# CATEGORY INDEX

## Herbs:

## Essential Oils:

## BATH

## Essential Oils:

## Home Remedies:

## BATH SALTS

## Essential Oils:

## DIET

### Ayurveda:

### Herbs:

### Home Remedies:

## DIFFUSER

### Essential Oils:

## DRINKS

### Ayurveda:

### Home Remedies:

## FOOT BATH

## GARGLE

## INFUSION

## INHALE

## LOTION

### Essential Oils:

## MASSAGE OIL

### Ayurveda:

### Herbs:

### Essential Oils:

### Home Remedy:

## MEDITATION

### Ayurveda:

### Home Remedies:

## OINTMENT

### Ayurveda:

### Herbs:

### Essential Oils:

## PASTE

### Ayurveda:

### Herbs:

**Home Remedies:**

## SACHET

**Herbs:**

**Home Remedies:**

## SALVE

### Herbs:

### Essential Oils:

### Home Remedies:

## SPRAY

### Essential Oils:

### Herbs:

### Home Remedies:

## SPRITZ

### Essential Oils:

## STEAM

**Ayurveda:**

**Essential Oils:**

## SYRUP

**Ayurveda:**

**Herbs:**

## TEA

**Ayurveda:**

**Herbs:**

## Home Remedies:

## WASH

### Herbs:

### Home Remedies:

## WRAP

## YOGA

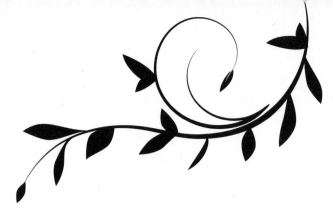

# ACKNOWLEDGMENTS

I wish first and foremost to thank Jane Dystel, my agent, of Dystel, Goderich & Bourret, for always believing in me. Jane makes every one of her authors feel as if they are her star. Thank you to Jane and the rest of the DG&B team for always having my back.

I want to thank everyone at Llewellyn that had a hand in making this book. This book is so special to me, and I dreamed of writing it for years. Angela Wix, my editor, I love your style, your no-nonsense approach, and how much you actually listen to what your authors want. I appreciate your wanting to include me in every aspect of this publishing process. Thank you from my soul to yours. There is a whole team of people at Llewellyn who work behind the scenes and make such beautiful things happen with my books. I want to thank each of them for their hard work and love of alternative healing. I want to extend a special wish of gratitude to Kat Sanborn, Becky Zins, Shira Atakpu, Lauryn Heineman, Andy Belmas, Anna Levine, and Melissa Mierva. You have all contributed much more to this book than I will ever be aware of. Thank you.

Vance: You were always my biggest supporter. Now you give your support and love to me in a much higher way. Thank you for continuing to be here for me from the Great Unknown. I miss you. I love you. I feel you.

Lin and Colleen: We've been through so many chapters of life together. We've shared untold hard, very hard, excruciating, exciting, wonderful, mundane, glorious, shocking, boring, exhilarating, horrible, and freeing experiences. I wouldn't want to journey through all of this with anyone else. How was I ever so lucky? How did I deserve you girls? The truth is that I have never deserved the love, respect, and what I have received from you both. I wish I could wrap the universe up and hand it to you. I love you. I love you. I love you.

To Chele and Thomas Michael J. Wagadorn Theodore Oliver Osburn Junior Gentles: I love you two insane people with all of my heart and soul. Chele … can you come help me put some stuff in the attic?

I would like to thank Amazon, Barnes & Noble, Baker & Taylor, Indigo Chapters in Canada, and Ingram for selling and promoting my books. Thank you.

To you believers in natural healing. Your emails, questions, support, and love of natural healing is what keeps me going and trying to improve with each book. I will continue to try and give you the books, knowledge, and support you want. I appreciate each and every one of you and will always strive to learn so that I can provide you with every new (or old) approach to healing safely and without any repercussions. Much healing to you!

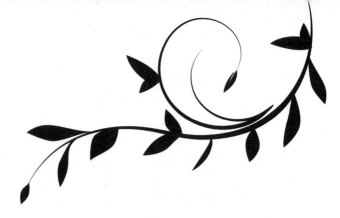

# INTRODUCTION

*Llewellyn's Book of Natural Remedies* provides a simple layout of recipes so that you can find what you need quickly and easily for your healing needs. Learning to heal naturally and effectively is paramount to our continuing health and well-being. There is not a one-thing-cures-all approach to natural or integrative healing methods. We learn from our ancestors, science, and a multitude of alternative healers. While essential oils may clear up your cold and help you sleep, herbs may help you on the path of emotional healing, and Ayurveda may help you to lose weight, get grounded, reduce stress, or heal a rash. It is a combination of these healing, life-long practices that make us healthy and knowledgeable. Home remedies from various cultures give us recipes that have been used for hundreds—and in some cases thousands—of years. They worked then, and they will work now.

*Llewellyn's Book of Natural Remedies* uses the integrative approach for minor everyday ailments. (More serious disorders should be seen by a physician or medical team for diagnosis and treatment.) Each of the ailments in this book can be treated myriad ways; four recipes follow each ailment. The recipes are divided into four categories: Ayurvedic treatments, herbs, essential oils, and home remedies. You can apply just one of the recipes or a combination of them to treat your current condition. This variety can open the door to treatments that you may not have realized were so beneficial.

## MY STORY

I used to sell insurance door-to-door. I liked the job, but physically it was too much for me. I had arthritis so bad in my neck, elbows, and shoulders, it was hard to carry the heavy leather bag of forms and books. My skin was split multiple times on my heels, and every step felt like I had glass grinding into the cuts. I had eczema all over my body in numerous outbreaks. I had not slept more than three hours a night for twenty years due to my restless leg syndrome. My lower back and other areas of my body were wracked with pain and inflammation due to autoimmune disorders. I was a physical wreck. Something had to give. I had to quit my job due to the physical hardships on my body. During this period of time, I was learning about herbs and had just started growing my own little herb garden.

As the years passed and my knowledge of diet, essential oils, and herbs grew, it became apparent to me that all the prescribed pills, creams, and topical ointments were not what was going to heal me, and some of them were furthering my illnesses. I needed to figure out why my body was doing what it was doing, and not just by treating it on the outside; I wanted to treat it from the inside, but without chemical medications. That's when I stumbled across a new (I thought) medical treatment called Ayurveda. It was exactly what I had been looking for. Ayurveda teaches us to use our mind, body, diet, and spirit to heal. Herbs, natural healing, and essential oils (my first loves) are a huge part of Ayurveda and are included in every facet of an Ayurvedic practitioner's life.

I learned to meditate, eat properly, exercise, and medicate according to the Ayurvedic tradition. Relieving anxiety and stress through Ayurvedic practices were paramount in my improving health, along with diet and detox. After several years of practice and learning to apply all of the herbs, essential oils, home remedies, and Ayurvedic teachings to myself, I improved in ways I never dreamed were possible. I went from envisioning my future in a wheelchair to having optimal physical, spiritual, and mental health, which was astonishing to me.

## SOME CAUTIONS

There are many tips and warnings pertaining to the usage of essential oils, herbs, and natural healing methods that I have listed for you. I cannot advise any of the recipes in this book as a treatment for any illness or disease, as I am not a physician or a diagnostician. Ensure through your doctor that you can incorporate these recipes into your care routine, especially if you are on any medications. You know yourself best. Do your research and learn about the products and services you are using.

All of the essential oils, herbs, or other natural remedies in this book come in varying strengths, potencies, and degrees of effectiveness. Research for yourself the brand or the amount you wish to use to ensure that you are getting the best product available. Ensure that you are using a safe essential oil before placing it on the skin, as essential oils can be very powerful or are sometimes made with other ingredients. You can ensure you are getting a good essential oil by several factors, such as price, ingredients, and integrity of the brand. You will want to check the ingredients to make sure that it is 100 percent essential oil. True essential oils are pricier than the oils made with byproducts. Experience with the oils is the truest way to learn which ones work and which ones do not. Have fun using the various brands and finding the one that works for you. I find uses for all of them, regardless of price or brand. The cheaper ones I use in my diffuser; the very good clinical-grade oils I use as medicine.

Never take any medicine internally, natural or chemical, without first checking with your physician and without checking the labels to determine whether or not you can take them internally. Many herbs, essential oils, and plants can have devastating consequences when used improperly or when combined with other medications or illnesses. Always store your essential oils, herbs, and other natural and chemical medications away from children. Storing essential oils and herbs in dark containers protects them from sunlight, which can lessen the potency of the product. Certain of these products can have fatal consequences when taken by children or adults. Never apply any medication to eyes, ears, mucus membranes, or sensitive areas without first checking with your physician.

Carrier oils are the oils that are used to mix with essential oils, thereby diluting them so that they will not burn or harm your skin. Essential oils are extremely concentrated and too potent to use most of them straight (also called "neat"). Blending and diluting them with a carrier oil can help to transport the oils to our skin and cells without damaging them. Carrier oil can be sesame, coconut, grapeseed, olive, jojoba, almond, or any oil you like that you feel will enhance the recipe you are making.

You can conduct a patch test with essential oils by mixing a drop of the essential oil with eight drops of carrier oil. Apply to your skin and leave on for twelve hours. Check at the end of twelve hours to ensure that your skin is not red, itching, blistered, or in any way harmed by the essential oil. If you do notice any skin irritation, then do not use that particular oil in any way.

Check with your doctor before using any of these recipes if you have any illness or are pregnant, nursing, trying to conceive, or have any medical issues at all.

These recipes are meant to be fun and healing. Follow all the rules and warnings to have the best results possible.

## AYURVEDA

Imagine going to your family doctor for a rash. He would probably give you a prescription for a topical ointment and tell you to come back in three months. The whole face-to-face visit is over in less than six minutes. Now imagine that you are going to an Ayurvedic practitioner. She may ask you any number of questions about your lifestyle that you feel don't in any way pertain to your rash—your diet, your job, your spirituality, or your home life. She might then suggest that you perform various activities that may sound strange to you—anything from wearing the color orange to following a vata diet. The whole visit can take two to three hours. The Ayurvedic practitioner treats you to increase your quality of life, not to temporarily heal your rash. And more importantly, she teaches you how you can treat yourself. This is the difference between Ayurveda and most Western medicine.

*Ayurveda* means "the science of life." It incorporates all aspects of life: diet, spiritual aspects, natural medicine, and how we actually live our lives on a day-to-day basis. Healing through Ayurvedic practices means not only healing yourself physically through diet, exercise, and medications, but healing mentally and spiritually as well.

Ayurvedic diets involve healthy and clean eating. While the first law of Ayurveda is to do no harm, vegetarianism is not a requirement to live Ayurvedically, but it is a healthier way to live. Ayurvedic practitioners believe that all illness begins in the gut. If you are eating improperly, it will catch up with you in the form of physical or mental illness. Processed foods are proven to be harmful to us, but in our fast-paced society, they are prevalent and easy to use. If you can try to eat natural and healthy foods at least 50 percent of the time, you will notice a huge difference in your body, mind, and soul. It truly is what we eat that determines our health for the rest of our lives. In most cases, your physical, mental, and spiritual conditions reflect your daily food intake.

Ayurvedic practitioners are often yogis who practice the physical and mental exercises of yoga. These poses, or asanas, can give such strengthening abilities to us physically, while soothing our minds at the same time. Breathing techniques make up a huge part of yoga and also help us to develop great endurance skills both physically and mentally. If you are not a practitioner of yoga, try a few classes, no matter your size, shape, religion, gender, or age. Buy a DVD or record some yoga shows and do them a couple times. Just get on the mat, and you will find that the benefits to your body, mind, and soul are immeasurable.

Ayurveda was derived from the Hindu religion, although Ayurveda itself is not a religion, but the science of life. You can adapt whatever religion you have to Ayurveda. Working on the soul's journey is a very important and necessary part of Ayurveda. How can we be healthy when our very base is shaky? We cannot. The base of all humanity is the spirit and soul. Work on your spiritual base daily, and watch your life become more solid, steady, and joyous. Ayurveda helps us learn about our individual spiritual journeys and how to strengthen our faith and our soul. Ayurveda uses meditation, prayer, introspection, and pure joy of the moment to teach us how insignificant we are as individuals and how together, as a whole, we can bring peace and contentment to the world. Helping others is a huge part of Ayurveda, and having a deep spiritual understanding of this can bring nothing but good to the earth—and that is with every religion. Whether Hindu, Buddhist, Christian, or Muslim, we can all deepen and develop our own personal spiritual path through Ayurvedic teachings.

When I first started writing this book, Ayurvedic recipes were the first recipes I wanted to include. Ayurveda is over four thousand years old and is the oldest form of medicine in the East. It's amazing how the ancient sages of India knew how important our mental and spiritual health was to our physical health. They knew that the plants put on this earth by the universe were meant for us to use to heal ourselves, and these plants still work today. The therapeutic properties in plants are what are copied and made chemically by scientists and turned into pharmaceutical drugs and used for medicine. Why use the copy of a plant when you can make a tea or an ointment using the actual properties from the plant? Ayurveda teaches us what foods, plants, and fruits we can use for certain ailments.

Keeping the doshas in balance is paramount in keeping the body, mind, and soul healthy the Ayurvedic way. The doshas are three different categories based on your personality, mentality, and physical appearance. Your doshas—either kapha, pitta, or vata—should be equal within you; however, most people have a primary dosha. Your dosha type is remarkably accurate in predicting your future illness, disease, and issues. Working on lowering your primary dosha and bringing up your secondary doshas is believed to lead to a much healthier and happier life. Ayurvedic practice focuses on balancing the doshas through diet, spiritual practice, various types of oils, herbs, colors, yoga, mantras, and gemstones. The list is endless on ways that you can incorporate natural healing methods to balance your doshas.

Kaphas are usually overweight, slow of speech, don't like to exercise, have oily hair and fair skin, and have low energy. Kaphas are generally very nonjudgmental and great listeners who are helpful to others. In Ayurveda it is believed that kaphas will eventually develop obesity, high blood pressure, heart issues, and sinus problems. Kaphas are thought to have too much water and are instructed to perform fire and air practices to balance their doshas.

Pittas are of medium build and quick to laughter but also have a temper and are quick to anger. Pittas have a strong sex drive, are often very charismatic, and are great speakers and debaters. Reducing the fire of pitta by adding more air and water is the way to keep pitta in check and reduce the chances of acquiring the pitta diseases. Pittas usually develop strokes, ulcers, digestion issues, and stress disorders.

Vatas are usually thin type A personalities with dry hair who walk fast, talk fast, and are usually leaders and great multitaskers. Ayurvedic practitioners believe that vatas will suffer from painful ailments as they age, such as arthritis, back pain, neck injuries, skin issues, and mental disorders. Vatas can suffer from anxiety and panic attacks and are generally fearful. Vatas are believed to have too much air so are instructed to perform grounding practices. Increasing your fire and water doshas will reduce your vata.

## Essential Oils

Oh, these little bottles of hidden treasures! Essential oils are like magic. How hundreds of pounds of flowers can be pressed, steamed, and turned into one ounce of liquid healing is almost supernatural. The medical benefits of these oils are phenomenal.

Essential oils date back thousands of years. Almost every ancient text has mention of at least one essential oil. Before pharmacies, drugstores, and hospitals, essential oils were used as very powerful medicine. Essential oils were more expensive than gold in ancient times. In some cases, these oils were used as money. Just think: when the three magi brought gifts to the baby Jesus, frankincense oil and myrrh oil were right up there with the gold.

I have worked with essential oils for many, many years. It's amazing to me how popular they have become in the last five years, primarily due to the home-based selling of essential oils through various companies. This has brought an explosion of essential oils into the hands of everyday people, drugstores, and even your local grocery stores. A lot of people currently have essential oils, but many of them don't know how to use them. This book is for you, as you will find easy-to-use recipes utilizing the most common essential oils.

## Herbs

Herbs are the universe's gift to us in order that we may heal ourselves. I am a certified herbalist who has grown and used over one hundred different species of herbs, and I believe that there is an herb for every illness. Including herbal recipes in this book was a no-brainer for me. I could not in good conscience write a book about natural healing remedies without including herbal recipes that can work for almost every ailment.

Herbs can be used in a variety of ways. There are plenty of books out there that teach us how to use herbs in both the culinary and medicinal worlds. Tinctures, ointments, balms, salves, teas, baths, and rubs are just a few of the ways that herbs can be manipulated into healing products. *Llewellyn's Book of Natural Remedies* shows you how to use the herbs in those capacities and much more.

When specifying the amounts of herbs to use in this book, dried herbs are the most common and plentiful, therefore dried herbs are the type of herbs listed in the recipes, unless otherwise specified. Fresh herbs contain a greater moisture content; you should use more fresh herbs in the place of dried herbs. Typically, 1½–2 times the amounts of fresh herbs are used in place of dried herbs.

Herbs were our first medicine. These plants, trees, shrubs, and flowers grow in almost every area of the world. People learned by trial and error which plants healed which diseases. Science copied the properties in these plants and developed medications for these same ailments. You can now make your own healing products cheaply and easily in your own home by reading, researching, and studying herbs.

All of the ancient medical texts are filled with depictions of the herbs that were used to end plagues, assist with childbirth, heal disease, and bring health and vitality to people of every culture. Herbs and the essential oils made from them are mentioned in the Holy Bible over one hundred times. Every country around the world has recipes for ailments made from herbs. It is surprising how many of the same recipes, especially for herbal teas, were used by every nation on earth. Herbs worked then, and they work now. Incorporating a few herbal concoctions into your medicine cabinet will ensure a healthier lifestyle for you and your family.

## HOME REMEDIES

Adam and Eve didn't have a local doctor to run to when they had a toothache or a crick in their neck. They had to figure out for themselves that a bite of peppermint soothed a stomachache or that a drop of aloe vera gel would make a wound heal faster. Home remedies are not just folk recipes from the 1800s; they are a vast collection of recipes for healing collected from ancient Egypt to modern herbalists, spanning thousands of years. Healing with everyday products from our kitchen seems too good to be true to us here in the West. We have spent the last one hundred years—our entire lives—running to the doctor every time we have an illness that lasts more than two days. We need to incorporate more natural healing into our daily lives and live less with chemical copies of medications, which often do more harm than good.

Reconnecting with nature and our forebears to learn how to heal ourselves again has recently become more popular. For years I have researched natural healing methods from around the world. While I do agree that for more serious ailments a medical team can get the best treatment and results for you, using natural products for minor ailments is often the healthier, and certainly a cheaper, way to go.

The home remedy recipes in this book contain a wide variety of treatments: herbs, gemstones, essential oils, color therapies, foods, mantras, liquids, tips, roots, prayers, yoga poses—the list is endless. During my research I looked for healing methods that were often used in more than one country and more than one time period with great results. When a treatment has been used for hundreds or even thousands of years, it's because it works! Oftentimes you may notice throughout the book that some ingredients and recipes seem to be repeated. The therapeutic properties in some of these ingredients work so well that they can be used for myriad complaints. Now you can use those same recipes to bring healing results for yourself.

Listening to the elders, healers, shamans, and sages from centuries past brings us a method of healing that was often kept secret from the general public. Safeguarding a healing treatment ensured that the healers had job security! *Llewellyn's Book of Natural Remedies* includes recipes that were thought to be magic and sorcery in their day.

A lot of the tips and hints for certain conditions seem like common sense, and they turn up over and over again in every culture throughout the world in medical journals, Vedic texts, and holy books. These tips include exercise, fresh air, reducing stress, healthy diet, adequate sleep, sunshine, hydration, and prayer. They may seem simple and redundant, but they are effective, and how often do we do the things that are best for us? When you see these lists of commonsense remedies, practice them. They are listed for a reason: they work.

I have used many of these recipes for most of my life. I enjoy healing with natural recipes and folk remedies. Knowing that I am drinking turmeric milk for a condition the same way Gandhi did is a thrill for me. Understanding that Shakespeare probably used thyme tea to cure his cough makes me so happy. Using these old home remedies is quick, cheap, and healing;

it's very useful information to have. I hope you enjoy learning about these ancient secrets and the power of healing. Knowing that you can use natural ingredients instead of pharmaceutically produced chemicals is a comfort and self-empowering thing indeed.

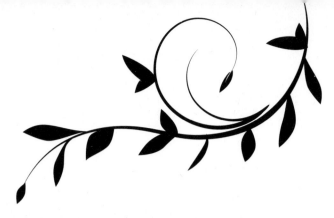

# WARNINGS AND
# THERAPEUTIC PROPERTIES

Following are lists of the most common herb and essential oil warnings and therapeutic properties for your general needs. Please heed all warnings. For the meaning of various therapeutic properties, please refer to the glossary.

• • • •
## HERBS

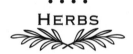

## AGRIMONY

**WARNINGS:** Agrimony can be phototoxic. It is unsafe to use if you are pregnant or breastfeeding or have diabetes. Before using agrimony, check with a healthcare provider prior to surgery.

**THERAPEUTIC PROPERTIES:** antibiotic, antibruising, antidiarrheal, anti-inflammatory, astringent, diuretic, febrifuge, styptic, tonic, vulnerary

## ALOE VERA

**WARNINGS:** Test for allergies. Not to be used orally if pregnant or breastfeeding. Not to be taken orally by children under the age of twelve. Should not be taken in large amounts internally.

**THERAPEUTIC PROPERTIES:** antibiotic, antifungal, anti-inflammatory, antiseptic, antitumor, antiviral, cicatrisant, cytophylactic, diuretic, immune boosting, laxative, vulnerary

## ANGELICA

**WARNINGS:** Angelica may raise or lower blood sugar, so those with heart disease, hypoglycemia, upcoming surgeries, diabetes, or blood pressure issues should not take angelica. Do not take if pregnant. Trying to abort with this herb has poisoned women.

**THERAPEUTIC PROPERTIES:** antibacterial, antinausea, antispasmodic, antiviral, carminative, diaphoretic, diuretic, emmenagogue, expectorant, febrifuge, pulmonary, stimulant, tonic

## ANISE

**WARNINGS:** Not to be used if you have a nervous disorder or are pregnant or nursing. Not for children under the age of six.

**THERAPEUTIC PROPERTIES:** antihysteric, anti-inflammatory, antinausea, antirheumatic, antiseptic, antispasmodic, aperitif, aphrodisiac, carminative, cordial, decongestant, digestive, diuretic, expectorant, nervine, sedative

## ARNICA

**WARNINGS:** Arnica should not be taken by diabetics or heart patients, as it is a blood thinner. Can cause depression and skin irritation and should not be taken with any other medication. Only take internally at the advice of a physician.

**THERAPEUTIC PROPERTIES:** antiarthritic, antibacterial, antibruising, anti-inflammatory, antispasmodic, gastro stimulant, hair restorative, immune stimulant, nervine, vasodilator, vulnerary

## ASTRAGALUS

**WARNINGS:** Consult your physician before taking astragalus with any other medication. There is a lack of evidence whether astragalus is harmful if pregnant or nursing. Not to be used on children.

**THERAPEUTIC PROPERTIES:** antibacterial, anti-inflammatory, antioxidant, circulatory stimulant, immune booster, vulnerary

## BASIL

**WARNINGS:** Do not use if pregnant or breastfeeding. Children under six years old or people with epilepsy should not use basil until more research has been completed.

**THERAPEUTIC PROPERTIES:** analgesic, antibacterial, antidepressant, antifungal, anti-infective, anti-inflammatory, antirheumatic, antiseptic, antispasmodic, antitussive, antiviral, carminative, cephalic, circulatory stimulant, diaphoretic, digestive, expectorant, galactogogue, nervine, purifying, relaxant, restorative, sedative, sudorific, tonic

## BEE BALM

**WARNINGS:** Children, people with thyroid issues, and pregnant or nursing women should not use bee balm. Can be phototoxic. May cause drowsiness.

**THERAPEUTIC PROPERTIES:** anticatarrhal, antinausea, aperitif, calming, carminative, decongestant, diaphoretic, febrifuge, relaxant, sedative

## BILBERRY

**WARNINGS:** Not to be taken by those about to have surgery, diabetics (as the lowering of blood sugar in conjunction with diabetic medicines could cause blood sugar to go too low), children, pregnant or nursing women, or those with epilepsy.

**THERAPEUTIC PROPERTIES:** antiarthritic, anticarcinogenic, anti-inflammatory, antioxidant, antiulcer, circulatory stimulant, cytophylactic, digestive, ophthalmic, vasodilator

## Black Cohosh

**WARNINGS:** Do not take if pregnant or nursing. Children should not use this. Long-term usage could increase chances of cancer, according to one study. No one with a chronic illness should take this herb.

**THERAPEUTIC PROPERTIES:** analgesic, antianxiety, antiarthritic, antibacterial, anti-inflammatory, antirheumatic, antispasmodic, digestive, emmenagogue, herbal estrogen, nervine, relaxant, sedative

## Black Horehound

**WARNINGS:** Should not be used by those with Parkinson's disease, psychotic disorders, or schizophrenia. Should not be used by children or pregnant or nursing women.

**THERAPEUTIC PROPERTIES:** anticatarrhal, antinausea, antispasmodic, astringent, cholagogue, nervine, pain relief, sedative, stimulant, vermifuge

## Black Pepper

**WARNINGS:** People with stomach issues such as ulcers, colitis, and diverticulitis should not use black pepper.

**THERAPEUTIC PROPERTIES:** analgesic, antiarthritic, antibacterial, anticarcinogenic, anticatarrhal, anti-inflammatory, antioxidant, antirheumatic, antiseptic, antispasmodic, aperient, carminative, cordial, decongestant, dental usages, diaphoretic, digestive, expectorant, neuralgic

## Blue Cohosh

**WARNINGS:** Do not take if pregnant or nursing. Anyone with heart disease, cancer, or any reproductive disease should avoid. Can cause birth defects or nausea.

**THERAPEUTIC PROPERTIES:** antiarthritic, antihysteric, antispasmodic, laxative

## BORAGE

**WARNINGS:** Do not take if pregnant or nursing. Do not take if you have a liver disorder or are taking blood thinners. Do not take two weeks before surgery.

**THERAPEUTIC PROPERTIES:** anticatarrhal, antidepressant, anti-inflammatory, antirheumatic, antiulcer, cordial, demulcent, diuretic, emollient, febrifuge

## BURDOCK ROOT

**WARNINGS:** Do not take if pregnant or nursing. Children under the age of two and people with liver disease should not use this.

**THERAPEUTIC PROPERTIES:** antibacterial, antifungal, bitter, diaphoretic, diuretic, emollient, laxative, tonic, vulnerary

## BUTTERBUR

**WARNINGS:** Do not take if pregnant or nursing. Do not take if you have any liver issues or ailments.

**THERAPEUTIC PROPERTIES:** diuretic, febrifuge, nervine, stimulant, tonic, vermifuge

## CALENDULA

**WARNINGS:** Do not take if pregnant or nursing.

**THERAPEUTIC PROPERTIES:** analgesic, anti-inflammatory, antipyretic, antispasmodic, aperient, diaphoretic, emmenagogue, expectorant, stimulant, vasodilator, vulnerary

## CARAWAY

**WARNINGS:** none

**THERAPEUTIC PROPERTIES:** analgesic, antibruising, antihysteric, aromatic, carminative, stimulant, stomachic

## CATNIP

**WARNINGS:** Occasional nausea by some people when taken in large quantities.

**THERAPEUTIC PROPERTIES:** antibruising, antihysteric, antispasmodic, carminative, diaphoretic, emmenagogue, nervine, sedative, stimulant, tonic

## CAYENNE

**WARNINGS:** Can cause inflammation of the mouth, throat, or rectum in some people.

**THERAPEUTIC PROPERTIES:** aromatic, carminative, febrifuge, rubefacient, stimulant

## CHAMOMILE

**WARNINGS:** Can cause allergies in some people. Should not be used during the first four months of pregnancy. Can be a skin irritant. Roman chamomile is less irritating than German chamomile. May cause drowsiness.

**THERAPEUTIC PROPERTIES:** analgesic, antiallergenic, antibiotic, antidepressant, antifungal, anti-infective, anti-inflammatory, antimicrobial, antineuralgic, antiphlogistic, antiseptic, antispasmodic, bactericidal, carminative, cholagogue, cicatrisant, cooling, digestive, emmenagogue, febrifuge, hepatic, nervine, sedative, stomachic, sudorific, tonic, vermifuge, vulnerary

GERMAN CHAMOMILE: analgesic, anti-allergenic, antibacterial, anti-inflammatory, antirheumatic, antispasmodic, digestive, fungicidal, sedative

ROMAN CHAMOMILE: analgesic, antiseptic, antispasmodic, digestive, sedative, respiratory distress

## CHICKWEED

WARNINGS: Can be toxic in large amounts.

THERAPEUTIC PROPERTIES: anticarcinogenic, anti-inflammatory, antiseptic, antitumor, demulcent, digestive, emollient, sedative

## CHICORY

WARNINGS: none

THERAPEUTIC PROPERTIES: anti-inflammatory, aperient, decongestant, diuretic, emollient, laxative, sedative, tonic

## CINNAMON

WARNINGS: Can cause dermatitis. Do not use on children. Should not be used if you are pregnant or suspect you are pregnant. Do not use during chemotherapy.

THERAPEUTIC PROPERTIES: antibacterial, anticlotting, antifungal, antimicrobial, astringent, carminative, cooling, stimulating

## CLEAVERS

WARNINGS: Has been known to cause a skin rash in some people.

THERAPEUTIC PROPERTIES: aperient, diuretic, tonic

## CLOVE

**WARNINGS:** Can cause dermatitis. Should not be used on children. Should not be used if you are pregnant or suspect you are pregnant. Clove is very strong and can burn the skin. Do not use in baths. Do not take with blood thinners.

**THERAPEUTIC PROPERTIES:** analgesic, antifungal, anti-inflammatory, antimicrobial, antirheumatic, antiseptic, antiviral, aphrodisiac, immune system stimulant, nervine, stimulant

## COMFREY

**WARNINGS:** Has been shown to have carcinogenic effects in research with rats. Do not take if pregnant or nursing. Do not take if you have liver disease or cancer. Never ingest comfrey.

**THERAPEUTIC PROPERTIES:** anticarcinogenic, anti-inflammatory, antirheumatic, antitussive, relieves heavy menstrual periods

## CORIANDER

**WARNINGS:** Can cause stomach issues. Should not be used if you are pregnant or suspect you are pregnant. Coriander is not safe if you have any kidney issues.

**THERAPEUTIC PROPERTIES:** Analgesic, aphrodisiac, antifungal, anti-inflammatory, antispasmodic, carminative, deodorant, detoxifier, digestive, fungicide, lipolytic, sedative, stomachic, vermifuge

## CRAMPBARK

**WARNINGS:** Relaxes the uterus. Should not be taken with other medications.

**THERAPEUTIC PROPERTIES:** antiasthmatic, antirheumatic, antispasmodic, nervine

## DANDELION

**WARNINGS:** Can cause upset stomach or skin rash.

**THERAPEUTIC PROPERTIES:** antirheumatic, aperient, detoxifier, diuretic, hepatic, stomachic, tonic

## DILL

**WARNINGS:** Can cause skin rash.

**THERAPEUTIC PROPERTIES:** antispasmodic, carminative, digestive, disinfectant, galactogogue, sedative, stomachic, sudorific

## DONG QUAI

**WARNINGS:** Not to be used if you are pregnant or nursing, have a heavy menstrual flow, or are on blood thinners.

**THERAPEUTIC PROPERTIES:** antidepressant, anti-inflammatory, antioxidant, circulatory stimulant, detoxifier

## ECHINACEA

**WARNINGS:** Do not take if pregnant or nursing. Do not take if you have asthma. Do not take with any other medications.

**THERAPEUTIC PROPERTIES:** antibiotic, antiseptic, antibacterial, antifungal, anti-inflammatory, antiviral, detoxifier, febrifuge, immune system booster, tonic

## ELDERFLOWER

**WARNINGS:** Uncooked berries from this plant are poisonous. Contains cyanide.

**THERAPEUTIC PROPERTIES:** Anticatarrhal, anti-inflammatory, antiviral, bronchial, and an immune strengthener. Elderflower is also believed to promote vivid dreams.

## EUCALYPTUS

**WARNINGS:** Do not use on children. Never take eucalyptus internally. Should be used with caution as some strong odors can trigger an asthma attack. Should not be used on the face or with any other medications. Do not use if you have high blood pressure.

**THERAPEUTIC PROPERTIES:** analgesic, antifungal, anti-inflammatory, antimicrobial, antirheumatic, antiseptic, antispasmodic, antiviral, bactericidal, decongestant, deodorant, diuretic, expectorant, mucolytic, stimulating

## EVENING PRIMROSE

**WARNINGS:** Use caution if pregnant or nursing.

**THERAPEUTIC PROPERTIES:** antiarthritic, anticoagulant, antispasmodic, astringent, hypertensive, liver regeneration

## EYEBRIGHT

**WARNINGS:** Has caused increased eye pressure and adverse effects in some people.

**THERAPEUTIC PROPERTIES:** anti-inflammatory, astringent

## FENNEL SEED

**WARNINGS:** Do not use if you are on birth control or if you have breast tumors or occasional clotting. Stop taking if you experience nausea or vomiting.

**THERAPEUTIC PROPERTIES:** antibruising, antiemetic, antiseptic, antispasmodic, aromatic, carminative, diaphoretic, digestive, diuretic, expectorant, galactogogue, hepatic, rubefacient, stimulant, stomachic

## FEVERFEW

**WARNINGS:** May cause mouth ulcers. Do not take if you are pregnant, nursing or taking blood thinners.

**THERAPEUTIC PROPERTIES:** anti-inflammatory, digestive, relaxant, vasodilator

## FLAXSEED

**WARNINGS:** Laxative. Do not use if nursing.

**THERAPEUTIC PROPERTIES:** anticatarrhal, anti-inflammatory, decongestant, demulcent, digestive, emollient, laxative

## GINGER

**WARNINGS:** Do not use if pregnant or nursing. Should not be taken by people on blood thinners. May cause stomach distress in heavy doses.

**THERAPEUTIC PROPERTIES:** antinausea, aphrodisiac, aromatic, carminative, digestive, rubefacient, stimulant

## GARLIC

**WARNINGS:** May cause rash in people allergic to garlic. Do not use if you are nursing or pregnant. Do not take if you also take blood thinners.

**THERAPEUTIC PROPERTIES:** antibacterial, anticarcinogenic, anticatarrhal, antifungal, anti-inflammatory, antimicrobial, antiseptic, antispasmodic, antiviral, carminative, cholagogue, detoxifier, diaphoretic, expectorant, hypotensive, rubefacient, stimulant, tonic, vulnerary

WARNINGS AND THERAPEUTIC PROPERTIES

## Ginkgo Biloba

**WARNINGS:** Do not take large amounts over an extended period of time. Do not take if you are on blood thinners or are having an upcoming surgery as ginkgo biloba causes bleeding.

**THERAPEUTIC PROPERTIES:** antiasthmatic, antibiotic, antidepressant, anti-infective, antioxidant, circulatory stimulant, decongestant, shock, nervine

## Ginseng

**WARNINGS:** Do not use if pregnant or nursing. Do not use if you have lupus. No one with a chronic condition should take this without first consulting a physician.

**THERAPEUTIC PROPERTIES:** aphrodisiac, stimulant, tonic, vasodilator

## Goldenseal

**WARNINGS:** Uterus stimulant. Do not take if pregnant. Do not use if you have high blood pressure. Do not take internally.

**THERAPEUTIC PROPERTIES:** antibacterial, antibiotic, anticatarrhal, antitumor, antiviral, astringent, cholagogue, digestive, emmenagogue, expectorant, hepatic, immune stimulant, laxative, tonic, vulnerary

## Gotu Kola

**WARNINGS:** Do not use if you have ever had cancer or take antidepressants or sedatives. Discontinue if rash develops. Do not use if pregnant or nursing.

**THERAPEUTIC PROPERTIES:** antibiotic, antidepressant, antirheumatic, anti-inflammatory, hypotensive, memory boosting, promotes circulation

## Green Tea

**WARNINGS:** Do not take if you are on blood thinners. Can cause allergic reactions.

**THERAPEUTIC PROPERTIES:** astringent, cephalic, nervine, stimulant

## Hawthorn

**WARNINGS:** Not to be taken if you have seizures or any heart condition. Do not take with any other medications.

**THERAPEUTIC PROPERTIES:** antidiarrheal, antispasmodic, circulation booster, digestive, sedative, stomachic

## Hibiscus

**WARNINGS:** Unsafe for pregnant women.

**THERAPEUTIC PROPERTIES:** antiallergenic, anticoagulant, antihaematomic, anti-inflammatory, antimicrobial, antiphlogistic, antiseptic, antitussive, cholagogue, cicatrisant, cytophylactic, diuretic, emollient, expectorant, febrifuge, fungicidal, hepatic, mucolytic, nervine, splenic

## Holy Basil

**WARNINGS:** Can cause low blood pressure. Should not be taken with blood thinners as basil can increase bleeding.

**THERAPEUTIC PROPERTIES:** aromatic, disinfectant

## Honeysuckle

**WARNINGS:** The berries are mildly poisonous.

**THERAPEUTIC PROPERTIES:** antibacterial, antifungal, enhances intuition

## HOPS

**WARNINGS:** Do not take with any other medication or if you have seizures.

**THERAPEUTIC PROPERTIES:** analgesic, antibacterial, antiseptic, astringent, digestive, hypnotic, immune stimulant, nervine, sedative

## HOREHOUND

**WARNINGS:** Do not take if you have any type of heart disease.

**THERAPEUTIC PROPERTIES:** antiasthmatic, antibruising, decongestant, expectorant, purgative, tonic, vulnerary

## HORSETAIL

**WARNINGS:** Can cause dermatitis.

**THERAPEUTIC PROPERTIES:** astringent, diuretic, vulnerary

## JUNIPER

**WARNINGS:** Do not use if you have any kidney disorders or take blood thinners.

**THERAPEUTIC PROPERTIES:** analgesic, antioxidant, antiseptic, astringent, cicatrisant, diuretic

## LAVENDER

**WARNINGS:** May cause drowsiness.

**THERAPEUTIC PROPERTIES:** Analgesic, antibiotic, anticonvulsive, antidepressant, antifungal, anti-infective, anti-inflammatory, antirheumatic, antiseptic, antispasmodic, antivenous, antiviral, bactericidal, cicatrisant, decongestant, deodorant, detoxifier, disinfectant, restorative, sedative, and tonic. Relieves irritability and nervous tension—great for test anxiety.

TRUE LAVENDER (LAVANDULA ANGUSTIFOLIA): The calming lavender. It can help restless babies, relieve insomnia, is great for burns and insect bites, relieve premenstrual syndrome, and can be effective against MRSA and tuberculosis.

SPIKE LAVENDER (LAVANDULA LATIFOLIA): The stimulating lavender. It can be used for chest congestion, sprains, stiff joints, and muscular pain. Do not give to children under the age of ten.

## Lemon Balm (Melissa)

**WARNINGS:** Do not use lemon balm if you are pregnant or nursing or have any thyroid issues. May cause drowsiness.

**THERAPEUTIC PROPERTIES:** Antidepressant, antihistaminic, antispasmodic, bactericidal, carminative, cordial, diaphoretic, emmenagogue, febrifuge, hypotensive, nervine, sedative, stomachic, sudorific, and tonic. *Melissa* can also be used as an insect repellant and is a good remedy to treat shock.

## Lemon Verbena

**WARNINGS:** none

**THERAPEUTIC PROPERTIES:** antispasmodic, carminative, febrifuge, sedative, stomachic

## Lemongrass

**WARNINGS:** Should not be taken during pregnancy or if you suspect you are pregnant.

**THERAPEUTIC PROPERTIES:** anti-inflammatory, antioxidant, fever reducer, immune booster, nervine, sedative, stomachic

## LINDEN

**WARNINGS:** none

**THERAPEUTIC PROPERTIES:** anti-anxiety, decongestant, nervine, sedative

## MAIDENHAIR FERN

**WARNINGS:** none

**THERAPEUTIC PROPERTIES:** anticatarrhal, decongestant, demulcent, emmenagogue, hepatic

## MARJORAM

**WARNINGS:** Should not be used during pregnancy or breastfeeding. Should not be used during depression.

**THERAPEUTIC PROPERTIES:** Analgesic, antiseptic, antispasmodic, aphrodisiac, antiviral, bactericidal, carminative, cephalic, cordial, diaphoretic, digestive, diuretic, emmenagogue, expectorant, fungicidal, hypotensive, laxative, nervine, sedative, stomachic, vasodilator, and vulnerary. Good for insomnia blends, aids with cramps, great to use during cold and flu season.

## MARSHMALLOW ROOT

**WARNINGS:** Not to be used with any other medication. Not to be used by diabetics.

**THERAPEUTIC PROPERTIES:** antiasthmatic, anti-inflammatory, demulcent, diuretic, emollient, vulnerary

## MILK THISTLE

**WARNINGS:** Can have severe side effects. Not to be taken with other medications. Can cause diarrhea. Violent reactions have occurred in some people.

**THERAPEUTIC PROPERTIES:** anticarcinogenic, anticatarrhal, antidepressant

## MULLEIN

**WARNINGS:** Not to be taken internally.

**THERAPEUTIC PROPERTIES:** antibacterial, anticatarrhal, anti-inflammatory, antiseptic, astringent, cephalic, decongestant, digestive (topical), emollient, sedative

## MUSTARD SEED

**WARNINGS:** none

**THERAPEUTIC PROPERTIES:** carminative, circulation stimulant, diuretic, emetic, rubefacient, stimulant, tonic

## NUTMEG

**WARNINGS:** A nutmeg overdose has been fatal in some people. Do not mix with other medications. Can have adverse effects such as nausea, seizures, and hallucinations. Do not take if you have any mental disorders, seizures, or neuralgic disorders.

**THERAPEUTIC PROPERTIES:** antinausea, aromatic, carminative, digestive, stimulant, stomachic

## OREGANO

**WARNINGS:** Do not use if you are pregnant or suspect you are pregnant. Do not use in baths as oregano is a skin irritant.

**THERAPEUTIC PROPERTIES:** analgesic, antiallergenic, antibacterial, antifungal, anti-inflammatory, antioxidant, antiparasitic, antiseptic, antispasmodic, antitoxic, antiviral, bactericidal, digestive, emmenagogue, fungicidal, stimulant, tonic

## OREGON GRAPE ROOT (POOR MAN'S GOLDENSEAL)

**WARNINGS:** Do not use while pregnant or nursing.

**THERAPEUTIC PROPERTIES:** antifungal, antimicrobial, digestive

## PASSIONFLOWER

**WARNINGS:** Not to be taken with blood thinners or sedatives.

**THERAPEUTIC PROPERTIES:** anti-anxiety, antihysteric, antispasmodic, cephalic, hypnotic, nervine, sedative

## PEPPERMINT

**WARNINGS:** Do not use if you are pregnant or suspect you are pregnant. Never put peppermint in the bath as it can cause skin irritation. Not to be used by small children. Peppermint cancels out any homeopathic remedies, so you should use one or the other.

**THERAPEUTIC PROPERTIES:** analgesic, anesthetic, antifungal, antigalactogogue, anti-infective, anti-inflammatory, antiphlogistic, antiseptic, antispasmodic, astringent, carminative, cephalic, cholagogue, cordial, decongestant, digestive, emmenagogue, expectorant, febrifuge, hepatic, invigorating, mucolytic, nervine, stimulant, stomachic, sudorific, vasoconstrictor, vermifuge

## PERIWINKLE

**WARNINGS:** none

**THERAPEUTIC PROPERTIES:** antiemetic, anti-inflammatory, astringent, emollient, laxative, tonic

## PLEURISY ROOT

**WARNINGS:** Do not take if you are pregnant or nursing. Do not give to children.

**THERAPEUTIC PROPERTIES:** anticatarrhal, antirheumatic, antispasmodic, carminative, cathartic, diaphoretic, expectorant, tonic

## PLANTAIN

**WARNINGS:** Causes allergic reactions in some people.

**THERAPEUTIC PROPERTIES:** anti-inflammatory, astringent, cephalic, diuretic, febrifuge, styptic, vulnerary

## RASPBERRY LEAF

**WARNINGS:** Not to be used by pregnant women. Speeds labor and delivery.

**THERAPEUTIC PROPERTIES:** astringent, cooling, febrifuge, stimulant, stomachic, vulnerary

## RED CLOVER

**WARNINGS:** Do not take if pregnant or nursing. Do not take if you have any blood disorder or are on blood thinners.

**THERAPEUTIC PROPERTIES:** anti-asthmatic, anticarcinogenic, anti-inflammatory, hormonal, tonic

## ROSE PETALS

**WARNINGS:** none

**THERAPEUTIC PROPERTIES:** antidepressant, antiphlogistic, antiseptic, antispasmodic, antiviral, aphrodisiac, astringent, bactericidal, cholagogue, cicatrisant, detoxifier, emmenagogue, hemostatic, hepatic, laxative, nervine, stomachic

## ROSEHIPS

**WARNINGS:** none

**THERAPEUTIC PROPERTIES:** anti-inflammatory, astringent, diuretic, laxative

## ROSEMARY

**WARNINGS:** Do not take if pregnant or nursing. Do not use if you have seizures, epilepsy, or high blood pressure. Children younger than four should not take rosemary.

**THERAPEUTIC PROPERTIES:** analgesic, antibacterial, anti-inflammatory, antirheumatic, antiseptic, antispasmodic, astringent, carminative, decongestant, disinfectant, diuretic, emmenagogue, restorative, stimulant, tonic

## SAGE

**WARNINGS:** If allergic, can cause mouth ulcers. Never use sage if you have high blood pressure or a seizure disorder.

**THERAPEUTIC PROPERTIES:** antibacterial, anticatarrhal, antifungal, anti-inflammatory, antimicrobial, antioxidant, antirheumatic, antiseptic, antispasmodic, cholagogue, choleretic, cicatrisant, detoxifier, digestive, disinfectant, emmenagogue, expectorant, febrifuge, laxative, stimulant

## SAVORY

**WARNINGS:** none

**THERAPEUTIC PROPERTIES**

SUMMER SAVORY: aromatic, carminative, cordial, digestive, expectorant

WINTER SAVORY: aromatic, digestive, stomachic

## SELF-HEAL

**WARNINGS:** Do not use while pregnant or nursing.

**THERAPEUTIC PROPERTIES:** antibiotic, antiseptic, antiviral, astringent, expectorant

## SHEEP'S SORREL

**WARNINGS:** none

**THERAPEUTIC PROPERTIES:** diaphoretic, diuretic, hepatic

## SKULLCAP

**WARNINGS:** Large amounts can cause adverse reactions. Do not take with sedatives. Do not take if you have diabetes or are pregnant or nursing.

**THERAPEUTIC PROPERTIES:** antirheumatic, antispasmodic, diuretic, nervine, sedative, tonic

## SLIPPERY ELM

**WARNINGS:** May cause allergic reactions.

**THERAPEUTIC PROPERTIES:** antidiarrheal, demulcent, digestive, emollient, stomachic

## SPEARMINT

**WARNINGS:** Do not use while pregnant or nursing.

**THERAPEUTIC PROPERTIES:** antiseptic, antispasmodic, carminative, cephalic, emmenagogue, expectorant, insecticide, nervine, restorative, stimulating, tonic

## ST. JOHN'S WORT

**WARNINGS:** Can be phototoxic after prolonged usage. Do not take with other antidepressants. Do not take if you have any mental disorders.

**THERAPEUTIC PROPERTIES:** antibacterial, antidepressant, anti-inflammatory, antiviral, astringent, cooling, immunostimulant, vermifuge

## TARRAGON

**WARNINGS:** People with a history of cancer should not take tarragon. Do not take when pregnant or nursing.

**THERAPEUTIC PROPERTIES:** Anti-inflammatory, antirheumatic, antiseptic, antispasmodic, aperitif, circulatory agent, digestive, deodorant, emmenagogue, stimulant, and vermifuge. Tarragon can also be used to stimulate the immune system and for mental stimulation.

## THYME

**WARNINGS:** Do not use on children. Do not use if you are pregnant or breastfeeding. Thyme should not be used in baths as it can be a skin irritant. People with high blood pressure should never use thyme.

**THERAPEUTIC PROPERTIES:** anticatarrhal, antidepressant, antimicrobial, antirheumatic, antiseptic, antispasmodic, astringent, bactericidal, bechic, cardiac, carminative, cephalic, cicatrisant, diaphoretic, digestive, diuretic, expectorant, hypertensive, insecticide, tonic, vermifuge, vulnerary

## TURMERIC

**WARNINGS:** Do not use if pregnant or nursing. Do not use if you have gallbladder or liver issues. May cause contact dermatitis.

**THERAPEUTIC PROPERTIES:** anti-inflammatory, aromatic, immune stimulant, stimulant

## UVA URSI

**WARNINGS:** Do not use if pregnant or nursing. Do not use if you have heart disease.

**THERAPEUTIC PROPERTIES:** antibacterial, antiseptic, diuretic, urinary

## VALERIAN

**WARNINGS:** Large amounts can cause adverse reactions. Do not take with other medications. Not enough information is known to be ensured of its safety during pregnancy or breastfeeding. May cause drowsiness.

**THERAPEUTIC PROPERTIES:** analgesic, antispasmodic, aromatic, calming, cicatrisant, nervine, sedative, stimulant, stomachic, tonic, tranquilizing

## VIOLET

**WARNINGS:** Do not use while pregnant or nursing.

**THERAPEUTIC PROPERTIES:** anti-inflammatory, aromatic, cephalic, laxative, sedative

## WHITE WILLOW BARK

**WARNINGS:** Not to be taken by children. Can cause stomach issues or allergic reactions. Not to be taken with other medications.

**THERAPEUTIC PROPERTIES:** analgesic, astringent, stimulant, tonic, vermifuge

## WILD CHERRY BARK

**WARNINGS:** Do not take if pregnant or nursing. Contains cyanide. Overdose is possible.

**THERAPEUTIC PROPERTIES:** anticatarrhal, astringent, decongestant, expectorant, sedative, tonic

## WILD LETTUCE

**WARNINGS:** none

**THERAPEUTIC PROPERTIES:** antispasmodic, hypnotic, nervine, sedative

## WITCH HAZEL

**WARNINGS:** Only use externally. Dilute for children.

**THERAPEUTIC PROPERTIES:** antibruising, anti-inflammatory, antitumor, antiseptic, astringent, sedative, styptic, tonic

## WORMWOOD

**WARNINGS:** Can cause epileptic seizures and liver damage. Do not take internally. Not to be used by pregnant or nursing women.

**THERAPEUTIC PROPERTIES:** antiemetic, aromatic, carminative, digestive (topical), febrifuge, nervine

## YARROW

**WARNINGS:** If you have hay fever, you may be allergic to yarrow. Do not use when pregnant or nursing. May cause headaches.

**THERAPEUTIC PROPERTIES:** anticatarrhal, anti-inflammatory, antirheumatic, antiseptic, antispasmodic, astringent, carminative, cicatrisant, diaphoretic, digestive, diuretic, emmenagogue, hemostatic, hepatic, hypotensive, stimulant, stomachic, tonic

## YELLOW DOCK

**WARNINGS:** Overdoses have resulted in death. Do not give to children. Do not take if pregnant or nursing. People with any diseases or any other medications should not take yellow dock.

**THERAPEUTIC PROPERTIES:** anticarcinogenic, antirheumatic, astringent, cytophylactic, emollient, laxative, stomachic, tonic

# ESSENTIAL OILS

Always conduct a patch test before using an essential oil. You can conduct a patch test by mixing a drop of the essential oil with eight drops of carrier oil. Apply to your skin and leave on for twelve hours. Check at the end of twelve hours to ensure that your skin is not red, itching, blistered, or in any way harmed by the essential oil. If you do notice any skin irritation, then do not use that particular oil in any way.

## ALOE VERA OIL

**WARNINGS:** No warnings discovered by this author. Please complete your own research before using this oil.

**THERAPEUTIC PROPERTIES:** analgesic, antibacterial, antifungal, anti-inflammatory, anti-irritant, antioxidant, antiviral, astringent, cicatrisant, cytophylactic, diuretic, emollient, vulnerary

## ANGELICA OIL

**WARNINGS:** Do not use if you are pregnant or nursing or think you may be pregnant. Do not use if you have diabetes, epilepsy, or seizures. Do not use on children. This oil is phototoxic and therefore should not be used before prolonged sun exposure.

**THERAPEUTIC PROPERTIES:** antispasmodic, carminative, detoxifier, diaphoretic, digestive, diuretic, emmenagogue, expectorant febrifuge, hepatic, holy, nervine, ritualistic, stimulant, stomachic, tonic

## ANISE OIL

**WARNINGS:** Anise oil should not be used for prolonged periods of time. Do not use if you are pregnant or nursing or think you may be pregnant.

**THERAPEUTIC PROPERTIES:** antiepileptic, antihysteric, antirheumatic, antiseptic, antispasmodic, aperient, carminative, cordial, culinary, decongestant, digestive, expectorant, insecticide, respiratory, sedative, stimulant, vermifuge

## ARNICA OIL

**WARNINGS:** Arnica oil should never be taken internally or applied to an open wound. Always use a carrier oil, such as jojoba, sesame, or grapeseed, with arnica oil. Arnica oil is known for causing skin issues and allergies in certain people.

**THERAPEUTIC PROPERTIES:** analgesic, antiarthritic, antibruising, anti-inflammatory

## BASIL OIL

**WARNINGS:** Always use a carrier oil, such as jojoba, sesame, or grapeseed, with basil oil as it can burn the skin. Do not use in bathwater. Do not use if you have epilepsy, seizures, or are pregnant or nursing.

**THERAPEUTIC PROPERTIES:** analgesic, antibacterial, antibiotic, antidepressant, anti-infective, anti-inflammatory, antiseptic, anti-spasmodic, antiviral, calming, carminative, culinary, digestive tonic, earaches, emmenagogue, holy, immune boosting, intestinal, ophthalmic, relaxant, restorative, ritualistic, general stimulant, stomachic

## BAY OIL

**WARNINGS:** Use sparingly for short durations of time.

**THERAPEUTIC PROPERTIES:** antibiotic, anti-neuralgic, antiseptic, anti-spasmodic, aperitif, emmenagogue, febrifuge, insecticide, sedative, stomachic

## BENZOIN OIL

**WARNINGS:** Should not be used in bathwater or in a diffuser as it is very thick and sticky and will adhere to skin. Always use a carrier oil (such as jojoba, sesame, or grapeseed) to help dilute the benzoin oil. Do not use on children.

**THERAPEUTIC PROPERTIES:** analgesic, antidepressant, anti-inflammatory, antirheumatic, antiseptic, astringent, calming, deodorant, carminative, cordial, disinfectant, diuretic, expectorant, euphoric, relaxant, sedative, vulnerary, warming

## BERGAMOT OIL

**WARNINGS:** Do not use if you are pregnant or nursing or think you may be pregnant. This oil is phototoxic and therefore should not be used before prolonged sun exposure. Always dilute with a carrier oil (such as jojoba, sesame, or grapeseed) before applying topically.

**THERAPEUTIC PROPERTIES:** analgesic, anti-anxiety, antibiotic, antidepressant, antiseptic, antispasmodic, aromatic, cicatrisant, deodorant, digestive, disinfectant, febrifuge, uplifting, vermifuge, vulnerary, weight reduction

## BIRCH OIL

**WARNINGS:** Birch oil is very potent. Always dilute with a carrier oil (such as jojoba, sesame, grapeseed, or your preference) before applying topically. Birch oil has had some severe allergies associated with its usage. Do not use if you are pregnant or nursing or think you may be pregnant.

**THERAPEUTIC PROPERTIES:** analgesic, antiarthritic, antibacterial, antidepressant, antifungal, anti-inflammatory, antirheumatic, antiseptic, antispasmodic, aromatic, astringent, cicatrisant, detoxifier, disinfectant, diuretic, febrifuge, germicide, insecticide, stimulant, tonic

## BLACK PEPPER OIL

**WARNINGS:** Do not use black pepper oil if you have any kidney issues as it can cause kidney damage.

**THERAPEUTIC PROPERTIES:** analgesic, antiarthritic, antibacterial, anticatarrhal, anti-inflammatory, antioxidant, antirheumatic, antiseptic, anti-spasmodic, aperient, carminative, culinary, diaphoretic, digestive, expectorant, respiratory, warming

## BLUE CYPRESS OIL (SEE CYPRESS OIL)

## BORAGE SEED OIL

**WARNINGS:** Borage seed oil can cause thinning of the blood. Do not take if you have upcoming tattoos or surgeries. Do not take borage seed oil if you have any liver issues.

**THERAPEUTIC PROPERTIES:** antiarthritic, anticatarrhal, antidepressant, anti-inflammatory, antirheumatic, antiulcer, cicatrisant, demulcent, diuretic, emollient, febrifuge, hormonal, purifier

## CAJUPUT OIL

**WARNINGS:** Please check with your physician before beginning a regimen of mixing cajuput oil with other medications. Do not use on children.

**THERAPEUTIC PROPERTIES:** analgesic, antifungal, antineuralgic, antioxidant, antiseptic, antispasmodic, bactericide, carminative, cosmetic, decongestant, diaphoretic, emmenagogue, expectorant, febrifuge, insecticide, respiratory, stimulant, sudorific, tonic, vermifuge, vulnerary

## CALENDULA OIL

**WARNINGS:** Do not use if you are pregnant or nursing or think you may be pregnant.

**THERAPEUTIC PROPERTIES:** antibruising, anticarcinogenic, anti-inflammatory, anti-itch, antipyretic, antispasmodic, antiulcer, cicatrisant, emmenagogue, menstrual cramps, stomachic, sudorific, tonic, vulnerary

## CAMPHOR OIL

**WARNINGS:** Do not use on open wounds or mucus membranes. Do not heat camphor oil. Do not use on children.

**THERAPEUTIC PROPERTIES:** anesthetic, anti-anxiety, anti-inflammatory, antineuralgic, antiseptic, antispasmodic, decongestant, disinfectant, insecticide, nervine, sedative, stimulant

## CARDAMOM OIL

**WARNINGS:** Cardamom has caused skin issues in some people.

**THERAPEUTIC PROPERTIES:** antimicrobial, antioxidant, antiseptic, antispasmodic, aphrodisiac, astringent, carminative, digestive, diuretic, expectorant, stimulant, stomachic

## CASSIA OIL

**WARNINGS:** Cassia oil should always be mixed with a carrier oil (such as jojoba, sesame, grapeseed, or your preference) before usage as it can cause burns due to its potency.

**THERAPEUTIC PROPERTIES:** antiarthritic, antidepressant, anti-diarrheal, antiemetic, antigalactogogue, antimicrobial, antirheumatic, antiviral, aromatic, astringent, carminative, circulatory, culinary, digestive, emmenagogue, febrifuge, immune booster, stimulant, uplifting, warming

## CEDARWOOD OIL

**WARNINGS:** Do not use on children. Cedarwood oil can terminate a pregnancy. Do not use if you are pregnant, nursing, think you may be pregnant, or are trying to conceive.

**THERAPEUTIC PROPERTIES:** antirheumatic, antiseborrheic, antiseptic, antispasmodic, aromatic, astringent, comforting, digestive, diuretic, emmenagogue, expectorant, fungicide, grounding, insecticidal, sedative, tonic

## CHAMOMILE OIL

**WARNINGS:** Chamomile oil can irritate the skin. Do not use if you are pregnant or nursing or think you may be pregnant.

**THERAPEUTIC PROPERTIES:** analgesic, antiallergenic, antibiotic, antidepressant, antifungal, anti-infective, anti-inflammatory, antimicrobial, antineuralgic, antiphlogistic, antiseptic, antispasmodic, aromatic, bactericidal, carminative, cholagogue, cicatrisant, comforting, cooling, deodorant, digestive, emmenagogue, febrifuge, hepatic, nervine, sedative, stomachic, sudorific, tonic, vermifuge, vulnerary, warming

GERMAN CHAMOMILE (MATRICARIA CHAMOMILLA):
analgesic, anti-allergenic, antibacterial, anticatarrhal,
anti-inflammatory, antiseptic, antispasmodic, carminative,
digestive, fungicidal, nervine, sedative

ROMAN CHAMOMILE (ANTHEMIS NOBILIS): antibiotic,
antidiuretic, anti-inflammatory, antimicrobial, antineuralgic,
antiphlogistic, antiseptic, antispasmodic, antitumor,
aromatic, bactericidal, carminative, cholagogue, digestive,
hepatic, tonic, sedative

## Cilantro Oil

WARNINGS: No warnings discovered by this author. Please
complete your own research before using this oil.

THERAPEUTIC PROPERTIES: analgesic, antispasmodic,
detoxifier, fungicidal, stomachic

## Cinnamon Bark Oil

WARNINGS: Cinnamon bark oil should not be used by those
undergoing cancer treatments such as chemotherapy or
radiation. This oil should always be diluted with a carrier oil
(such as jojoba, sesame, grapeseed, or your preference) as it can
cause significant burns to the skin if undiluted. Do not use in
baths. Do not use if you are pregnant or nursing or think you
may be pregnant.

THERAPEUTIC PROPERTIES: analgesic, antibacterial,
anticarcinogenic, anticlotting, antifungal, antimicrobial,
antioxidant, aromatic, astringent, carminative, cooling,
culinary, digestive, hypotensive, insecticide, uplifting,
stimulating

## CITRUS OILS

**WARNINGS:** These oils are phototoxic and therefore should not be used before prolonged sun exposure.

**THERAPEUTIC PROPERTIES:** antibacterial, antitoxic, antiviral, aromatic, astringent, circulatory, culinary, detoxifier, germicidal, uplifting

## CLARY SAGE OIL

**WARNINGS:** Do not use with low blood pressure or if you are hypoglycemic. Can cause drowsiness, so it's better to not drive or operate heavy machinery while using this oil. Do not use if you are pregnant or nursing or think you may be pregnant.

**THERAPEUTIC PROPERTIES:** anticonvulsive, antidepressant, antiseptic, antispasmodic, aphrodisiac, aromatic, astringent, bactericidal, calming, carminative, deodorant, digestive, emmenagogue, euphoric, hormones, hypotensive, nervine, opthalmic, restorative, sedative, soothing, stomachic, tonic, uterine, vulnerary

## CLEMATIS OIL

**WARNINGS:** Do not ingest.

**THERAPEUTIC PROPERTIES:** antispasmodic, antisyphilis, antiulcer, cicatrisant, nervine, stomachic, varicose veins, vulnerary, vulnerary

## CLOVE OIL

**WARNINGS:** A natural blood thinner, do not take clove oil if you are taking blood thinners or are scheduled for an upcoming tattoo or surgery. Clove oil is very thick and strong; do not use in diffuser or in baths. Always dilute with a carrier oil (such as jojoba, sesame, grapeseed, or your preference). Do not use if you are pregnant or nursing or think you may be pregnant.

**THERAPEUTIC PROPERTIES:** analgesic, anesthetic, anti-inflammatory, antifungal, antimicrobial, antirheumatic, antiseptic, antiviral, aphrodisiac, aromatic, bactericidal, carminative, culinary, insecticide, stimulant

## COMFREY OIL

**WARNINGS:** Do not take internally. Do not take if you have a liver disease or a serious disease such as cancer. Do not use if you are pregnant or nursing or think you may be pregnant.

**THERAPEUTIC PROPERTIES:** anti-inflammatory, antibronchitis, antirheumatic, antiulcer, diarrhea, heavy menstrual periods, persistent cough, respiratory, vulnerary

## CORIANDER OIL

**WARNINGS:** Do not take if you have any kidney issues or if you are pregnant or nursing or think you may be pregnant.

**THERAPEUTIC PROPERTIES:** analgesic, antirheumatic, antispasmodic, aphrodisiac, aromatic, carminative, culinary, deodorant, detoxifier, diarrhea, digestive, flatulence, fungicide, hemorrhoids, hernia, lipolytic, loss of appetite, nausea, stimulant, stomachic, stomach spasms, upset stomach

## COSMOS OIL

**WARNINGS:** No warnings discovered by this author. Please complete your own research before using this oil.

**THERAPEUTIC PROPERTIES:** antibacterial, antioxidant, aromatic, insecticidal

## CYPRESS OIL

**WARNINGS:** Do not use on varicose veins. Do not use if you are pregnant or nursing or think you may be pregnant.

**THERAPEUTIC PROPERTIES:** anti-infective, anti-inflammatory, antiparasitic, antirheumatic, antiseptic, antispasmodic, astringent, decongestant, deodorant, diuretic, hormone issues, restorative, vasoconstrictor

## DILL OIL

**WARNINGS:** No warnings discovered by this author. Please complete your own research before using this oil.

**THERAPEUTIC PROPERTIES:** antiarthritic, antimicrobial, antioxidant, antispasmodic, carminative, culinary, digestive, disinfectant, galactogogue, sedative, stomachic, sudorific

## ECHINACEA OIL

**WARNINGS:** No warnings discovered by this author. Please complete your own research before using this oil.

**THERAPEUTIC PROPERTIES:** analgesic, anti-allergen, anti-infective, anti-inflammatory, antibacterial, antibiotic, antioxidant, antirheumatic, antiviral, immune booster, respiratory, urinary

## EUCALYPTUS OIL

**WARNINGS:** Eucalyptus can trigger asthma attacks and should never be used in conjunction with other medications, on the face, on children, or by people with high blood pressure.

**THERAPEUTIC PROPERTIES:** analgesic, anti-inflammatory, antibacterial, antifungal, antimicrobial, antiseptic, antispasmodic, antiviral, aromatic, bactericidal, decongestant, deodorant, diuretic, expectorant, mucolytic, stimulating, tonic, vulnerary

## FENNEL OIL

**WARNINGS:** Fennel oil should not be used if you have seizures, cancer, kidney issues, or hormone problems. Do not use if you are pregnant or nursing or think you may be pregnant.

**THERAPEUTIC PROPERTIES:** analgesic, anti-inflammatory, antibruising, antidepressant, antiemetic, antiseptic, antispasmodic, diaphoretic, digestive, diuretic, laxative, opthalmic, rubefacient, stimulant

## FIR OIL

**WARNINGS:** Do not use if you are pregnant or nursing or think you may be pregnant.

**THERAPEUTIC PROPERTIES:** analgesic, anti-infective, anti-inflammatory, antibacterial, antioxidant, antiseptic, aromatic, calming, deodorant, detoxifier, grounding, respiratory, warming

## FRANKINCENSE OIL

**WARNINGS:** Do not use if you are pregnant or nursing or think you may be pregnant.

**THERAPEUTIC PROPERTIES:** analgesic, anti-inflammatory, antiasthmatic, antiseptic, astringent, calming, carminative, cicatrisant, cytophylactic, digestive, disinfectant, diuretic, emmenagogue, expectorant, grounding, holy, ritualistic, sedative, spiritual, tonic, uplifting, uterine, vulnerary

## GARLIC OIL

**WARNINGS:** Do not give garlic oil to babies. Do not use if you are pregnant or nursing or think you may be pregnant.

**THERAPEUTIC PROPERTIES:** anti-hypertensive, antibacterial, anticarcinogenic, anticatarrhal, antidandruff, antifungal, antimicrobial, antioxidant, antiseptic, antiviral, carminative, culinary, detoxifier, expectorant, hypotensive, vasodilator

## GERANIUM OIL

**WARNINGS:** Do not use if you are pregnant or nursing or think you may be pregnant. Do not use if you have low blood sugar or skin issues. May cause insomnia.

**THERAPEUTIC PROPERTIES:** analgesic, anti-anxiety, anti-inflammatory, antibacterial, antidepressant, antifungal, antiseptic, aromatic, astringent, bactericidal, cicatrisant, culinary, cytophylactic, deodorant, diuretic, hemostatic, styptic, tonic, vermifuge, vulnerary

## GINGER OIL

**WARNINGS:** Do not use ginger oil if you are on blood thinners or have sensitive skin or gallstones.

**THERAPEUTIC PROPERTIES:** analgesic, anti-inflammatory, antiemetic, antioxidant, antiseptic, antispasmodic, bactericidal, carminative, cephalic, culinary, expectorant, febrifuge, laxative, rubefacient, stimulant, stomachic, sudorific, tonic

## GINGKO BILOBA OIL

**WARNINGS:** No warnings discovered by this author. Please complete your own research before using this oil.

**THERAPEUTIC PROPERTIES:** anti-infective, anti-inflammatory, antiasthmatic, antidepressant, antioxidant, circulatory, decongestant, energizer, memory booster, nervine, stimulant

## GINSENG OIL

**WARNINGS:** No warnings discovered by this author. Please complete your own research before using this oil.

**THERAPEUTIC PROPERTIES:** anti-anxiety, anti-inflammatory, antioxidant, aphrodisiac, appetite suppressant, enhances circulation, immune booster, stimulant, tonic, vasodilator

## GRAPEFRUIT OIL

**WARNINGS:** This oil is phototoxic and therefore should not be used before prolonged sun exposure. Do not use if you have a skin condition as it can irritate the skin.

**THERAPEUTIC PROPERTIES:** anti-anxiety, antidepressant, antioxidant, antiseptic, appetite reduction, aromatic, astringent, culinary, disinfectant, diuretic, energizer, lymphatic, stimulant, tonic

## HELICHRYSUM OIL (IMMORTELLE, EVERLASTING)

**WARNINGS:** Do not use with blood thinners. Do not use on children. Do not use if you are pregnant or nursing or think you may be pregnant.

**THERAPEUTIC PROPERTIES:** analgesic, anti-inflammatory, antiallergenic, antibruising, anticoagulant, antidepressant, antifungal, antimicrobial, antiseptic, antispasmodic, antitussive, antiviral, cicatrisant, expectorant, hepatic, holy, ritualistic, tonic

## HIBISCUS OIL

**WARNINGS:** Do not use if you are pregnant or nursing or think you may be pregnant.

**THERAPEUTIC PROPERTIES:** anti-inflammatory, antiallergenic, anticarcinogenic, anticoagulant, antihaematomic, antimicrobial, antiphlogistic, antiseptic, antitussive, aromatic, cholagogue, cicatrisant, cytophylactic, diuretic, dye, emollient, expectorant, febrifuge, fungicidal, hepatic, hypertensive, immune booster, nervine, splenic, weight reduction

## HOLLY OIL

**WARNINGS:** No warnings discovered by this author. Please complete your own research before using this oil.

**THERAPEUTIC PROPERTIES:** antirheumatic, circulation, digestive, hypertensive, protection, purgative

## HONEYSUCKLE OIL

**WARNINGS:** No warnings discovered by this author. Please complete your own research before using this oil.

**THERAPEUTIC PROPERTIES:** antibacterial, antifungal, aromatic, culinary, intuition enhancer

## HYSSOP OIL

**WARNINGS:** Do not use if you are pregnant or nursing or think you may be pregnant. Do not use if you have a seizure disorder or high blood pressure. Do not mix with other medications.

**THERAPEUTIC PROPERTIES:** anti-infective, antiarthritic, antibruising, antirheumatic, antiseptic, antispasmodic, aromatic, astringent, carminative, cicatrisant, digestive, diuretic, emmenagogue, expectorant, febrifuge, holy, hypertensive, nervine, ritualistic , stimulant, sudorific, tonic, vermifuge, vulnerary

## JASMINE OIL

**WARNINGS:** Do not use if you are pregnant or nursing or think you may be pregnant.

**THERAPEUTIC PROPERTIES:** anti-anxiety, antidepressant, antiseptic, antispasmodic, aphrodisiac, aromatic, cicatrisant, emmenagogue, expectorant, galactogogue, parturient, respiratory, ritualistic, sedative, spiritual, uterine

## JUNIPER BERRY OIL

**WARNINGS:** Do not take for extended periods of time. Do not take if you have kidney issues. Do not mix with other medications. Do not use if you are pregnant or nursing or think you may be pregnant.

**THERAPEUTIC PROPERTIES:** anti-infective, anti-inflammatory, antifatigue, antirheumatic, antiseptic, antispasmodic, antitoxic, astringent, carminative, circulatory stimulant, detoxifier, diuretic, energizer, rubefacient, stimulating, stomachic, sudorific, tonic, vulnerary

## LAVENDER OIL

**WARNINGS:** No warnings discovered by this author. Please complete your own research before using this oil.

**THERAPEUTIC PROPERTIES:** analgesic, anti-anxiety, anti-infective, anti-inflammatory, antibiotic, anticonvulsive, antidepressant, antifungal, antimicrobial, antirheumatic, antiseptic, antispasmodic, antivenous, antiviral, aromatic, bactericidal, calming, cicatrisant, decongestant, deodorant, detoxifier, disinfectant, hypotensive, nervine, restorative, sedative, tonic, tranquilizing

TRUE LAVENDER (LAVANDULA ANGUSTIFOLIA): analgesic, antidepressant, calming, holy, hormonal, ritualistic, spiritual, vulnerary

SPIKE LAVENDER (LAVANDULA LATIFOLIA): analgesic, antiarthritic, aromatic, decongestant , expectorant, insecticidal, stimulant

LAVANDIN (LAVANDULA ×INTERMEDIA): anti-infective, antidepressant, calming, cicatrisant, expectorant, nervine, sedative

## Lemon Oil

**WARNINGS:** This oil is phototoxic and therefore should not be used before prolonged sun exposure. Do not use if you are pregnant or nursing or think you may be pregnant. Can cause skin irritation.

**THERAPEUTIC PROPERTIES:** antispasmodic, aromatic, astringent, culinary, detoxifier, germicidal, immune booster, tonic, uplifting

## Lemon Balm Oil (See Melissa Oil)

## Lemon Thyme Oil

**WARNINGS:** Do not use if you are pregnant or nursing or think you may be pregnant.

**THERAPEUTIC PROPERTIES:** anti-anxiety, antiaging, antiasthmatic, antispasmodic, aromatic, calming, culinary, decongestant, immune boosting, relaxant

## Lemongrass Oil

**WARNINGS:** Do not use if you are pregnant or nursing or think you may be pregnant.

**THERAPEUTIC PROPERTIES:** analgesic, anti-inflammatory, antidepressant, antioxidant, antipyretic, aromatic, astringent, bactericidal, calming, culinary, febrifuge, fungicidal, immune boosting, mood enhancer, nervine, sedative, stomachic, uplifting

## Lime Oil

**WARNINGS:** Do not use if you are pregnant or nursing or think you may be pregnant. This oil is phototoxic and therefore should not be used before prolonged sun exposure.

**THERAPEUTIC PROPERTIES:** anti-infective, antiseptic, antiviral, aperitif, aromatic, astringent, bactericidal, culinary, disinfectant, febrifuge, hemostatic, respiratory, restorative, tonic

## Linden Blossom Oil

**WARNINGS:** No warnings discovered by this author. Please complete your own research before using this oil.

**THERAPEUTIC PROPERTIES:** anti-anxiety, anti-inflammatory, anticarcinogenic, calming, diuretic, expectorant, hypertensive, immune booster

## Lotus Oil

**WARNINGS:** Not enough known about use during pregnancy. Avoid if pregnant or nursing. No other warnings discovered by this author.

**THERAPEUTIC PROPERTIES:** aphrodisiac, aromatic, astringent, calming, chakras, emmenagogue, expectorant, holy, hypnotic, hypotensive, meditative, ritualistic, sedative, tranquilizing, vasodilator

## Mandarin Oil

**WARNINGS:** This oil is phototoxic and therefore should not be used before prolonged sun exposure.

**THERAPEUTIC PROPERTIES:** antibacterial, antiseptic, antispasmodic, antiviral, aromatic, bactericidal, balancing, calming, circulatory, cytophylactic, detoxifier, digestive, expectorant, hepatic, nervine, relaxant, sedative, stomachic, tonic

## MANUKA OIL

**WARNINGS:** No warnings discovered by this author. Please complete your own research before using this oil.

**THERAPEUTIC PROPERTIES:** anti-anxiety, anti-inflammatory, antiallergenic, antibacterial, antidandruff, antifungal, antihistaminic, calming, cicatrisant, cytophylactic, deodorant, nervine, vulnerary

## MARJORAM OIL

**WARNINGS:** Do not use if you are taking blood thinners. Do not use if you have depression. Do not use if you are pregnant or nursing or think you may be pregnant.

**THERAPEUTIC PROPERTIES:** analgesic, antiseptic, antispasmodic, antiviral, aphrodisiac, bactericidal, carminative, cephalic, cordial, culinary, diaphoretic, digestive, diuretic, emmenagogue, expectorant, fungicidal, holy, hypotensive, laxative, nervine, ritualistic, sedative, spiritual, stomachic, tranquilizing, vasodilator, vulnerary

## MELALEUCA OIL (TEA TREE OIL)

**WARNINGS:** No warnings discovered by this author. Please complete your own research before using this oil.

**THERAPEUTIC PROPERTIES:** anti-infective, anti-inflammatory, anti-itch, antiallergenic, antibacterial, antibiotic, antifungal, antimicrobial, antiparasitic, antiseptic, antiviral, balsamic, cicatrisant, decongestant, dental, emollient, expectorant, fungicide, immune stimulant, insecticide, respiratory, stimulant, sudorific, vaginal infections, vasodilator, vulnerary

## MELISSA OIL (LEMON BALM OIL)

**WARNINGS:** Do not take if you have thyroid issues. Do not use if you are pregnant or nursing or think you may be pregnant. May cause drowsiness.

**THERAPEUTIC PROPERTIES:** antibacterial, antidepressant, antihistaminic, antispasmodic, bactericidal, bronchial, carminative, cordial, diaphoretic, emmenagogue, febrifuge, hypotensive, insect repellant, nervine, sedative, stomachic, sudorific, tonic, vulnerary

## MYRRH OIL

**WARNINGS:** Do not use if you are pregnant or nursing or think you may be pregnant.

**THERAPEUTIC PROPERTIES:** analgesic, anti-inflammatory, antibacterial, anticatarrhal, antifungal, antimicrobial, antiseptic, antispasmodic, astringent, carminative, cicatrisant, circulatory, diaphoretic, emollient, expectorant, holy, immune stimulant, mucolytic, revitalizing, ritualistic, sedative, stimulant, stomachic, tonic, vulnerary

## MYRTLE OIL

**WARNINGS:** Do not use internally or if you have any pulmonary issues. Do not use on children. Do not use if you are pregnant or nursing or think you may be pregnant.

**THERAPEUTIC PROPERTIES:** anti-inflammatory, antimicrobial, antiseptic, astringent, deodorant, digestive (topical), expectorant, nervine, respiratory, sedative, uplifting

## NEEM OIL

**WARNINGS:** Do not use internally. Do not use on children. Do not use if you are pregnant or nursing or think you may be pregnant. Do not use if you have autoimmune disorders, multiple sclerosis, rheumatoid arthritis, any liver issues, or any pulmonary issues.

**THERAPEUTIC PROPERTIES:** anti-inflammatory, anti-parasitic, antibacterial, anticarcinogenic, antifungal, antioxidant, antiulcer, antiviral, dental, detoxifier (topical)

## NEROLI OIL

**WARNINGS:** Neroli can be a skin irritant for some people. Do not use on children.

**THERAPEUTIC PROPERTIES:** anti-anxiety, anti-infective, antidepressant, antiseptic, antispasmodic, aphrodisiac, aromatic, bactericidal, carminative, cephalic, cicatrisant, cordial, cytophylactic, deodorant, digestive, disinfectant, emollient, sedative, tonic

## NIAOULI OIL

**WARNINGS:** No warnings discovered by this author. Please complete your own research before using this oil.

**THERAPEUTIC PROPERTIES:** analgesic, anti-inflammatory, antimalarial, antimicrobial, antirheumatic, antiseptic, bactericidal, balsamic, cicatrisant, decongestant, expectorant, febrifuge, insecticide, respiratory, stimulant, urinary, vermifuge, vulnerary

## ORANGE OIL

**WARNINGS:** This oil is phototoxic and therefore should not be used before prolonged sun exposure.

**THERAPEUTIC PROPERTIES:** anti-inflammatory, antibacterial, antidepressant, antimicrobial, antiseptic, antispasmodic, aphrodisiac, aromatic, carminative, cholagogue, culinary, diuretic, immune stimulant, sedative, tonic

## OREGANO OIL

**WARNINGS:** Do not apply directly to skin, such as in the bathtub, as it can cause rashes or burns. Always dilute oregano oil with a carrier oil (such as jojoba, sesame, grapeseed, or your preference). Do not use if you are pregnant or nursing or think you may be pregnant.

**THERAPEUTIC PROPERTIES:** analgesic, anti-infective, anti-inflammatory, antiallergenic, antiarthritic, antibacterial, anticarcinogenic, antifungal, antioxidant, antiparasitic, antiseptic, antispasmodic, antitoxic, antiviral, bactericidal, culinary, digestive, disinfectant, emmenagogue, fungicidal, respiratory, stimulant, tonic

## Oregon Grape Root Oil

**WARNINGS:** Do not use if you are pregnant or nursing or think you may be pregnant.

**THERAPEUTIC PROPERTIES:** anti-infective, antifungal, antimicrobial, antiulcer, aromatic, cleansing, detoxifier, digestive, skin issues, spiritual, stomachic

## Palmarosa Oil

**WARNINGS:** No warnings discovered by this author. Please complete your own research before using this oil.

**THERAPEUTIC PROPERTIES:** anti-anxiety, antiarthritic, antirheumatic, antiseptic, antiviral, bactericidal, cytophylactic, digestive, febrifuge, hydration balm, nervine, skin issues

## Patchouli Oil

**WARNINGS:** Patchouli oil should not be taken by people with any eating disorders.

**THERAPEUTIC PROPERTIES:** anti-inflammatory, antidepressant, antimicrobial, antiphlogistic, antiseptic, aphrodisiac, aromatic, astringent, bactericidal, calming, cicatrisant, cytophylactic, deodorant, diuretic, emollient, febrifuge, fixative, fungicide, grounding, insecticide, nervine, sedative, tonic

## PEPPERMINT OIL

**WARNINGS:** Peppermint oil can cause skin irritation, so do not use in the bath. Never use peppermint oil with prescribed medications. Do not use if you are pregnant or nursing or think you may be pregnant.

**THERAPEUTIC PROPERTIES:** analgesic, anesthetic, anti-inflammatory, antifungal, antigalactogogue, anti-infective, antiphlogistic, antiseptic, antispasmodic, aromatic, astringent, carminative, cephalic, cholagogue, cicatrisant, cordial, culinary, decongestant, digestive, emmenagogue, emollient, expectorant, febrifuge, hepatic, invigorating, mucolytic, nervine, nervousness, respiratory problems, stimulant, stomachic, sudorific, vasoconstrictor, vermifuge, vertigo

## PERU BALSAM OIL

**WARNINGS:** Do not use if you are pregnant or nursing or think you may be pregnant. Do not use if you have allergies or kidney issues. Do not take internally.

**THERAPEUTIC PROPERTIES:** anti-infective, anti-inflammatory, antifungal, antiparasitic, antiseptic, aromatic, calming, grounding, respiratory, vulnerary

## PETITGRAIN OIL

**WARNINGS:** No warnings discovered by this author. Please complete your own research before using this oil.

**THERAPEUTIC PROPERTIES:** antidepressant, antiseptic, antispasmodic, aromatic, balancing, calming, cicatrisant, cosmetic, deodorant, nervine, sedative, uplifting

## PINE OIL

**WARNINGS:** Do not use if you have sensitive skin. Do not use if you have high blood pressure. Do not use if you are pregnant or nursing or think you may be pregnant.

**THERAPEUTIC PROPERTIES:** analgesic, antibacterial, antioxidant, antirheumatic, antiseptic, aromatic, boosts metabolism, culinary, decongestant, detoxifier, diuretic, energizing, relaxant, rubefacient, urinary

## PINK GRAPEFRUIT OIL

**WARNINGS:** No warnings discovered by this author. Please complete your own research before using this oil.

**THERAPEUTIC PROPERTIES:** anticarcinogenic, antioxidant, antiseptic, detoxifier, energizer, purifier, tonic, weight control, weight reduction

## POPPY OIL

**WARNINGS:** No warnings discovered by this author. Please complete your own research before using this oil.

**THERAPEUTIC PROPERTIES:** analgesic, anticarcinogenic, antispasmodic, astringent, diaphoretic, expectorant, hypnotic, sedative

## RAVENSARA OIL

**WARNINGS:** No warnings discovered by this author. Please complete your own research before using this oil.

**THERAPEUTIC PROPERTIES:** analgesic, anti-inflammatory, antiallergenic, antibacterial, antidepressant, antifungal, antimicrobial, antioxidant, antiperspirant, antiseptic, antispasmodic, antitumor, antiviral, aphrodisiac, aromatic, carminative, cicatrisant, disinfectant, diuretic, expectorant, nervine, relaxant, tonic

## ROMAN CHAMOMILE OIL (SEE CHAMOMILE OIL)

## ROSE OIL

**WARNINGS:** Do not use if you are pregnant or nursing or think you may be pregnant.

**THERAPEUTIC PROPERTIES:** antiarthritic, anticarcinogenic, antidepressant, antiphlogistic, antiseptic, antispasmodic, antiviral, aphrodisiac, aromatic, astringent, bactericidal, cholagogue, cicatrisant, culinary, detoxifier, emmenagogue, hemostatic, hepatic, laxative, nervine, ritualistic, stomachic, uterine tonic

## ROSEMARY OIL

**WARNINGS:** Do not use if you have seizures, high blood pressure, or epilepsy. Do not use if you are pregnant, nursing, think you may be pregnant, or are trying to get pregnant. Do not use on children.

**THERAPEUTIC PROPERTIES:** analgesic, anti-inflammatory, antiaging, antibacterial, anticarcinogenic, antioxidant, antirheumatic, antiseptic, antispasmodic, aromatic, astringent, carminative, circulatory, culinary, decongestant, digestive, disinfectant, diuretic, immunity booster, memory enhancer, restorative, stimulant, tonic

## SAGE OIL

**WARNINGS:** Do not use if you have high blood pressure or any type of seizures.

**THERAPEUTIC PROPERTIES:** anti-inflammatory, antiaging, antibacterial, antifungal, antimicrobial, antioxidant, antiseptic, antispasmodic, aromatic, cholagogue, choleretic, cicatrisant, culinary, detoxifier, digestive, disinfectant, emmenagogue, expectorant, febrifuge, focus, immune booster, laxative, positivity, stimulant

## SANDALWOOD OIL

**WARNINGS:** Do not use if you have any kidney issues. Sandalwood oil can cause allergic skin reactions.

**THERAPEUTIC PROPERTIES:** anti-inflammatory, antifungal, antiphlogistic, antiseptic, antispasmodic, aphrodisiac, astringent, calming, carminative, cicatrisant, decongestant, disinfectant, diuretic, emollient, expectorant, grounding, harmonizing, hypotensive, insecticide, memory booster, memory enhancer, mental clarity, relaxing, sedative, tonic

## SESAME OIL

**WARNINGS:** No warnings discovered by this author. Please complete your own research before using this oil.

**THERAPEUTIC PROPERTIES:** anti-anxiety, anti-inflammatory, antiaging, anticarcinogenic, antidepressant, antifungal, antioxidant, antirheumatic, cosmetic, culinary, digestive, grounding, purifying

## SPEARMINT OIL

**WARNINGS:** Do not take internally. Do not use if you are pregnant or nursing or think you may be pregnant.

**THERAPEUTIC PROPERTIES:** anti-anxiety, antibacterial, antifatigue, antiseptic, antispasmodic, aromatic, calming, carminative, cephalic, circulatory, culinary, emmenagogue, expectorant, hormonal, immune boosting, insecticide, nervine, relaxing, respiratory, restorative, stimulating, stomachic, tonic

## SPIKENARD OIL

**WARNINGS:** Do not use if you are pregnant or nursing or think you may be pregnant.

**THERAPEUTIC PROPERTIES:** anti-anxiety, anti-inflammatory, antibacterial, antibiotic, antidepressant, antifungal, antioxidant, deodorant, digestive, grounding, holy, laxative, meditative, respiratory, rituals, sedative, spiritual, uterine, vasoconstrictor

## SPRUCE OIL

**WARNINGS:** Do not use if you are pregnant or nursing or think you may be pregnant. Do not take if you have any type of heart condition or asthma.

**THERAPEUTIC PROPERTIES:** anti-infective, anti-inflammatory, antiarthritic, antimicrobial, antirheumatic, antispasmodic, aromatic, disinfectant, expectorant, grounding, immune system stimulant, mentally invigorating, respiratory, strengthens nervous system, vulnerary

## ST. JOHN'S WORT OIL

**WARNINGS:** Do not mix with other medications unless under supervision of your prescribing doctor. Watch for side effects. This oil is phototoxic and therefore should not be used before prolonged sun exposure.

**THERAPEUTIC PROPERTIES:** anti-anxiety, anti-inflammatory, antiarthritic, antidepressant, antineuralgic, antioxidant, antirheumatic, astringent, cicatrisant, cooling, decongestant, hormonal, immunostimulant, vermifuge

## SWEET ORANGE OIL

**WARNINGS:** Use caution when giving to children and do not use for long periods of time. This oil is phototoxic and therefore should not be used before prolonged sun exposure.

**THERAPEUTIC PROPERTIES:** anti-anxiety, anti-inflammatory, anticarcinogenic, anticoagulant, antidepressant, antimicrobial, antiseptic, antispasmodic, aromatic, carminative, cholagogue, cicatrisant, circulative, culinary, detoxifier, digestive, diuretic, energizing, germicidal, relaxing, restorative, stomachic, tonic

## TANGERINE OIL

**WARNINGS:** This oil is phototoxic and therefore should not be used before prolonged sun exposure.

**THERAPEUTIC PROPERTIES:** anti-infective, antibacterial, anticarcinogenic, antifungal, antiseptic, antispasmodic, antiulcer, aromatic, calming, culinary, cytophylactic, detoxifier, restorative, sedative, stomachic, tonic, vulnerary, weight reduction

## TARRAGON OIL

**WARNINGS:** Do not use if you are pregnant or nursing or think you may be pregnant.

**THERAPEUTIC PROPERTIES:** anti-inflammatory, antifatigue, antirheumatic, antiseptic, antispasmodic, aperitif, aromatic, balancing, circulatory agent, deodorant, detoxifier, digestive, emmenagogue, hormonal, stimulant, stomachic, vermifuge

## TEA TREE OIL (MELALEUCA)

**WARNINGS:** No warnings discovered by this author. Please complete your own research before using this oil.

**THERAPEUTIC PROPERTIES:** anti-infective, anti-inflammatory, anti-itch, antiallergenic, antibacterial, antibiotic, antifungal, antimicrobial, antiparasitic, antiseptic, antiviral, balsamic, cicatrisant, decongestant, dental, emollient, expectorant, fungicide, immune stimulant, insecticide, respiratory, stimulant, sudorific, vaginal infections, vasodilator, vulnerary

## THYME OIL

**WARNINGS:** Do not use in the bathtub as it will cling to skin and burn. This oil is too thick to use in a diffuser and may harm your diffuser. Do not use on children. Do not use if you have high blood pressure. Do not use if you are pregnant or nursing or think you may be pregnant.

**THERAPEUTIC PROPERTIES:** anti-infective, anti-inflammatory, antimicrobial, antirheumatic, antiseptic, antispasmodic, aromatic, bactericidal, bechic, bronchial, cardiac, carminative, cicatrisant, culinary, digestive, diuretic, emmenagogue, expectorant, hypertensive, immunostimulant, insecticide, restorative, stimulant, tonic, vermifuge

## VALERIAN OIL

**WARNINGS:** This oil does not have enough evidence to present as safe to use during pregnancy or breastfeeding or trying to conceive. I would advise to not use during those times. Do not combine with other medications.

**THERAPEUTIC PROPERTIES:** analgesic, anti-anxiety, antidepressant, antispasmodic, calming, cicatrisant, hormonal, nervine, positivity, rituals, sedative, stomachic, tranquilizing

## VANILLA OIL

**WARNINGS:** No warnings discovered by this author. Please complete your own research before using this oil.

**THERAPEUTIC PROPERTIES:** anticarcinogenic, antidepressant, antioxidant, aphrodisiac, aromatic, culinary, febrifuge, hormonal, relaxant, sedative, tranquilizing

## VETIVER OIL

**WARNINGS:** Do not take consistently for long periods of time.

**THERAPEUTIC PROPERTIES:** anti-inflammatory, anticarcinogenic, antidepressant, antioxidant, antiseptic, aphrodisiac, calming, cicatrisant, cooling, febrifuge, relaxant, sedative, tranquilizing

## VITAMIN E OIL

**WARNINGS:** Do not ingest.

**THERAPEUTIC PROPERTIES:** antiaging, antiarthritic, anticarcinogenic, antifatigue, antioxidant, antiperspirant, cicatrisant, emollient, preservative

## WHEAT GERM OIL

**WARNINGS:** Do not use if you have celiac disease.

**THERAPEUTIC PROPERTIES:** antiaging, antioxidant, bactericidal, cell regenerator, emollient

## WHITE FIR OIL

**WARNINGS:** No warnings discovered by this author. Please complete your own research before using this oil.

**THERAPEUTIC PROPERTIES:** analgesic, anti-infective, anti-inflammatory, antiaging, anticarcinogenic, antioxidant, antirheumatic, antiseptic, aromatic, cardiovascular, detoxifier, expectorant, respiratory, ritualistic, spiritual, weight reduction

## WILD ORANGE OIL

**WARNINGS:** No warnings discovered by this author. Please complete your own research before using this oil.

**THERAPEUTIC PROPERTIES:** antimicrobial, antioxidant, antirheumatic, antiseptic, aromatic, carminative, cicatrisant, cleanser, culinary, detoxifier, digestive, diuretic, energizer, febrifuge, hypotensive, immune booster, purifying, stomachic, uplifting

## WINTERGREEN OIL

**WARNINGS:** There are many warnings about wintergreen oil. It is a very effective arthritis pain reliever, but do not use for extended periods of time. Ensure through your physician that it is safe to use wintergreen oil with your prescribed medications. Watch for side effects. Do not give to children. Do not use if you are pregnant or nursing or think you may be pregnant.

**THERAPEUTIC PROPERTIES:** analgesic, anodyne, antiarthritic, antirheumatic, antiseptic, antispasmodic, aromatic, astringent, calming, carminative, culinary, diuretic, emmenagogue, spiritual, stimulant, stress reduction, warming

## YARROW OIL

**WARNINGS:** Has been known to cause headaches in some people. Do not use if you are pregnant or nursing or think you may be pregnant.

**THERAPEUTIC PROPERTIES:** anti-inflammatory, antirheumatic, antiseptic, antispasmodic, astringent, carminative, cicatrisant, circulative, diaphoretic, digestive, expectorant, febrifuge, hemostatic, hypotensive, nervine, stomachic, styptic, tonic, vulnerary

## YLANG-YLANG OIL

**WARNINGS:** Do not use if you are on blood thinners or have high blood pressure. May cause headaches. Watch for side effects. Can cause skin allergies in some people. Do not use if you are pregnant or nursing or think you may be pregnant.

**THERAPEUTIC PROPERTIES:** anti-infective, antidepressant, antiseborrheic, antiseptic, aphrodisiac, aromatic, balancing, calming, cicatrisant, euphoric, hormonal, hypotensive, meditative, nervine, relaxant, sedative, tonic, tranquilizing

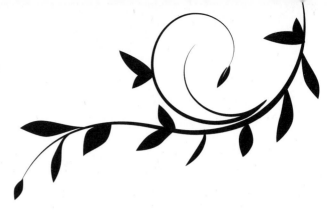

# CONDITIONS AND RECIPES

These ailments are the most common and easily treatable conditions that plague some member of our families every day. Knowing that you can follow a few guidelines and warnings and then make these recipes in your own home can be such an empowering feeling. We love to make ourselves and our loved ones feel as healthy as they can. Incorporating these recipes into their lives will ensure that your safe and chemical-free healing alternatives will be passed down for many generations to come.

• • • •

## ABDOMINAL PAIN

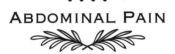

Abdominal pain can be caused by cramping, bloating, gas, allergies, or a myriad of reasons. If pain persists or fever is present, a medical diagnosis should be sought immediately. People have used natural remedies for pain in the digestive tract for thousands of years. These particular recipes have helped millions of people overcome abdominal pain.

### AYURVEDA: *Ayurvedic Candy*

In Ayurveda it is common to treat abdominal pain with plants, herbs, and oils. Ginger is used quite commonly and is good for other parts of your body as well. Therapeutic properties in ginger include analgesic, antiemetic, antispasmodic, bactericidal, carminative, laxative, stomachic, and tonic components, all of which help heal a painful tummy.

1 TABLESPOON GRATED GINGER

1 TEASPOON HONEY

4 DROPS LEMON OR LIME JUICE

Mix ingredients together to form a sticky ball. Cut ball into four pieces. Eat a piece every few hours until you no longer have abdominal pain. Store remainder, wrapped in plastic, in the refrigerator for up to three days.

## HERB: *Abdominal Herbal Tea*

This is one of the oldest and most comforting recipes in the world. Chamomile tea not only assists with easing abdominal pain, but it also can help you get a peaceful night's sleep. The therapeutic properties of chamomile include analgesic, antiallergenic, anti-inflammatory, and antispasmodic agents.

1 CUP WATER

1 TEASPOON CHAMOMILE FLOWERS

Bring water to a boil, then add herbs. Remove from heat, cover, and steep for six to eight minutes. Strain and, if desired, add sweetener of choice. Compost or discard herbs.

## ESSENTIAL OIL: *Peppermint Inhale*

Peppermint has been hailed for centuries as the go-to plant for abdominal distress. Peppermint contains anesthetic, anti-inflammatory, antispasmodic, carminative, and emmenagogue properties to get stomach pains to cease.

1 DROP PEPPERMINT OIL

Apply oil to palm of hand, oil inhaler, or tissue. Bring the essential oil close to your nostrils and inhale the aroma deeply. This process sends the properties straight to your brain, and the effects are immediate. You can complete this procedure three to four times a day.

## HOME REMEDY: *Home Healing Diets*

Oftentimes the way we eat can have a significant impact on our health. Abdominal stress may be a sign that the quality or the quantity of food you are eating is not agreeing with you.

Try to eat natural, healthy foods and stay away from greasy, spicy, sugary foods for a few days. You may like the way you feel so much that you won't ever want to go back to eating unhealthy again. That being said, allergies and intolerances of certain foods affect us more than we know.

Trying to eat healthy can be a daunting task, but the health and benefits that you will gain are extraordinary. Incorporate as many fibrous vegetables into your diet as possible, staying away from starchy vegetables such as potatoes and corn.

• • • •

# ABSCESS

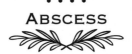

Abscesses can be anywhere in or on the body. An abscess is an infection in a localized area. Medical treatment to determine the diagnosis and stages of treatment should be a priority. The point of infection may become so infected or swollen that medical intervention may be needed to lance the site and prevent the infection from spreading, which can be detrimental. Abscesses are often accompanied by fever, chills, and fatigue. People have turned to anti-inflammatory herbs, oils, and plants to reduce the pain and rid the body of abscesses for millenniums.

## AYURVEDA: *Flax Paste*

Making a thick paste to apply to external abscesses is the most common way to treat them. This blend helps the pus to release and drains the abscess.

½ TEASPOON DRIED, GROUND ECHINACEA FLOWERS

½ TEASPOON GROUND FLAXSEED

½ TEASPOON WATER

Combine the ingredients in a small bowl to make a thick paste. Apply the paste to the abscess and allow to dry. You may cover with a bandage to protect clothing and furniture. Leave mixture on for several hours or overnight. Rinse and reapply as needed. Discard any remaining paste.

## HERB: *Echinacea Pain-Relieving Herbal Tea*

An infection is nothing to ignore. Medical professionals can prescribe antibiotics to bring much-needed healing. This recipe will provide temporary pain relief due to its antibiotic, antiseptic, anti-inflammatory, and febrifuge properties.

**1 CUP WATER**

**2 TEASPOONS ECHINACEA**

Bring water to a boil, then add herbs. Remove from heat, cover, and steep for six to eight minutes. Strain and, if desired, add sweetener of choice. Compost or discard herbs.

## ESSENTIAL OIL: *Peppermint Oil Pain Beater*

Peppermint has analgesic, anesthetic, anti-infective, anti-inflammatory, and antiseptic properties to bring healing and pain reduction to your abscess.

**2 DROPS PEPPERMINT OIL**

**5 DROPS SESAME OIL OR ANOTHER CARRIER OIL**

Combine oils and apply around the abscess, making sure to not get it inside if the skin is broken. Do not apply to open wounds, genitals, mucus membranes, or sensitive areas.

## HOME REMEDY: *Pain Management Meditation Remedy*

Many people are able to escape pain temporarily through meditation. Try this meditation exercise for at least five minutes. This technique is taught in pain management classes throughout the world.

Find a nice quiet place where you can relax without being disturbed. Sit in a comfortable spot and cross your legs, if possible. Bring your hands, palms up, to rest on your knees. Close your eyes as you breathe slowly and deeply. Sit with a straight back and long neck. Breathe in, hold the breath for a couple seconds, and slowly breathe out.

Imagine that you are in a garden where you can walk among the flowers and plants. Visualize the peace and happiness that each and every plant brings to you. Imagine that you can inhale the aroma of the flowers as you bend down to smell them and take in their beauty, all the while concentrating on your deep breathing as you relax your shoulders and jaw. When your mind begins to wander, gently coax it back to your garden.

Meditation has been proven to be an effective way to battle chronic pain. Repeat this practice as needed until you can see your dentist or doctor.

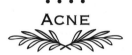

# ACNE

Acne is a skin condition often occurring throughout puberty. Scarring can occur if not treated. The oil glands under the skin become blocked and then infected. Dermatologists can offer many treatments for treating acne, but they are often very expensive. Essential oils, herbs, Ayurvedic treatments, and home remedies have been used for centuries to put an end to acne. Ensure that you complete an allergy test if it is the first time you are using one of these essential oils.

## AYURVEDA: *Herbal Derma Infusion*

Basil is good for much more than making our pasta taste delicious! Basil's therapeutic properties include antibacterial, antibiotic, anti-infective, anti-inflammatory, and antiseptic, and it is also a very good tonic. This infusion will help your skin glow and get rid of any skin issues that you have. Sip infusion slowly throughout the day or take a spoonful at a time through the course of a few hours.

**1 CUP FILTERED WATER**

**4 TEASPOONS BASIL LEAVES**

Bring water to a boil, then add herbs. Remove from heat, cover, and steep for twenty to thirty minutes. Strain and, if desired, add sweetener of choice. Compost or discard herbs. Drink slowly throughout the day, one teaspoonful at a time. Discard any remainder at the end of the day. Repeat for three days.

## HERB: *Herbal Detoxifier*

Burdock and dandelion root contain vulnerary, antibacterial, emollient, anti-fungal, detoxifying, and tonic therapeutic properties. Cleaning out your system is a good way to get glowing, healthy skin.

1 CUP WATER

1 TEASPOON BURDOCK ROOT

1 TEASPOON DANDELION ROOT

Bring water to a boil, then add herbs. Remove from heat, cover, and steep for six to eight minutes. Strain and, if desired, add sweetener of choice. Compost or discard herbs.

## ESSENTIAL OIL: *Acne Spray*

Lemon contains astringent and detoxifying components to help you get rid of that acne quickly. Use this spray daily after you clean your face in your normal fashion. This is the recipe that we use often in our family for both teenage and menopausal outbreaks.

15 DROPS LEMON OIL

2 OUNCES FILTERED WATER

1 TEASPOON WITCH HAZEL

Combine the ingredients into a spray bottle and shake well. Lightly spray the outbreak area, ensuring you close your eyes and mouth, and allow to air-dry. Do not spray into eyes, genitals, open wounds, mouth, or mucus membranes. Shake well before each use. Store in a cool, dark area for up to six months.

## HOME REMEDY: *Spot-On Natural Remedy*

Garlic contains antiseptic, antimicrobial, antibacterial, antifungal, detoxifying, anti-inflammatory, and vulnerary healing properties. This old-fashioned remedy has been used for years and years.

1 GARLIC CLOVE

Cut the garlic clove in half and, using the "wet" side, run it over the outbreak area several times. Allow to air-dry. Repeat process several times daily until your acne clears up. Discard any garlic at the end of the day.

· · · ·

# ADHD (ATTENTION DEFICIT HYPERACTIVITY DISORDER)

When a person is unable to focus for any length of time, unable to control emotions and actions, and has abnormal physical activity, this may be diagnosed as ADHD. This is often controlled with medications by the family physician. Essential oils, herbs, Ayurvedic treatments, and home remedies can alleviate some of the issues associated with ADHD. You can use these recipes or make your own combinations of oils to try. Ensure that you are not allergic to any particular ingredients by doing a patch test twenty-four hours before beginning to apply the components of the recipes (see page 4).

## AYURVEDA: *Mood Techniques*

Yoga, meditation, and exercise are some excellent ways to calm a person suffering from ADHD. The lack of focus and concentration can be controlled for longer and longer periods of time as the person learns to quiet the mind and relax into poses and meditation. These tips incorporate some of the balancing techniques that have been used in Ayurveda forever to calm and quiet the mind and body.

- Practice soothing and calming yoga poses. The corpse pose is the best for calming the mind and the body. Lay flat on your back. Relax the feet and allow them to drop naturally into position. Rest hands at the sides, palms up. Close your eyes, slowly breathe in and out, and think only peaceful thoughts. Placing a wet, cool cloth over the eyes with a drop of lavender oil on it will help with relaxation. Imagine you are an ice cube melting in the sun, and keep the corpse position for five minutes.

- What you eat *is* what you are. Try a diet of healthy, non-sugary, non-breaded foods. Ghee is an important ingredient in Ayurveda and in controlling ADHD. Ghee is available at most health-food stores—grass-fed is best—but it is also easy to make yourself. Try cooking chicken in ghee and serving with warm vegetables. Do not eat cold foods or sandwiches. Eat foods without preservatives or artificial coloring.

- One of the most effective ways to calm the mind and bring balance and peace to the soul is with a walk in nature. Allow yourself to run and play, wander aimlessly, and to have fun and to let your interest be piqued while exploring the outdoors.

- Massage the entire body from neck to toes with massage oil. This is relaxing and grounding. Use either olive oil or sesame oil for an added boost to calm and balance. Follow up with a warm bath or shower.

- Try turning off all electronics one hour before bedtime. Reading a book is recommended, as is meditation, caffeine-free herbal teas, simple yoga stretches, and praying. Making a routine out of bedtime can reward everyone exponentially.

### HERB: *ADHD Tea*

These herbs contain calming, focusing and soothing properties. A cup of this tea will relax even the most hyperactive of people. Usually taken before bedtime or rest.

**1 CUP WATER**

**½ TEASPOON CHAMOMILE FLOWERS**

**½ TEASPOON LEMON BALM LEAVES**

**½ TEASPOON VALERIAN ROOT**

Bring water to a boil, then add herbs. Remove from heat, cover, and steep for ten minutes. Strain and, if desired, add sweetener of choice. Compost or discard herbs.

### ESSENTIAL OIL: *Calm Me Down Massage Oil*

Receiving a massage is a gift in and of itself. Add these essential oils with their sedative properties and you will have your patient so calm and relaxed that focusing on attention to detail will come naturally and peacefully.

**8 DROPS LEMON BALM (MELISSA) OIL**

**8 DROPS VETIVER OIL**

**5 DROPS VITAMIN E OIL**

**1 OUNCE SESAME OR OLIVE OIL**

Mix ingredients in a glass container and lightly massage the desired area, such as the back or the soles of the feet. Keep essential oil mixture away from open wounds, mucus membranes, genitals, eyes, and sensitive areas. Repeat application as needed. Store unused portion in a glass jar with a tight-fitting lid in a cool, dark area for up to three months.

## HOME REMEDY: *ADHD Apple Cider Vinegar Remedy*

While it seems too simple to even fathom, apple cider vinegar has been used for ages to help heal internally what comes out physically. In other words, calming the digestive tract can calm the mind. Apple cider vinegar has the same effect as probiotics on the gastro system. Using this simple remedy can help a person to heal from the inside out.

### 1–2 TEASPOONS APPLE CIDER VINEGAR

### ½ CUP WATER

Mix the ingredients together and drink before you have your biggest meal of the day. The taste may not be good, so sometimes adding honey when first starting the routine will get a person used to the taste, and then the honey can be reduced until simply taking vinegar in water is the norm.

• • • •

# AGE SPOTS (LIVER SPOTS)

Age spots are caused by the sun and the ultraviolet rays that attack our skin cells. Many people have lightened those spots exponentially with these treatments. These recipes from around the world can help to even out or alleviate age spots and give you back your glowing skin.

## AYURVEDA: *Cumin Infusion Rub*

Middle Eastern women have used this recipe for generations with great results. They are in the sun most of the time, and this rub helps even out their skin tone.

### 1 CUP WATER

### 2 TEASPOONS CUMIN SEEDS

Bring water to boil, then steep cumin seeds for fifteen to thirty minutes. Cool. Dab on the age spot repeatedly throughout the day for several days. You can soak a bandage in the mixture and apply to spot if it's in a good place for adhering a bandage. Keep remainder in a jar with a tight-fitting lid in the refrigerator for up to three days.

## HERB: *Dandelion Herbal Tea*

Dandelions are good for so many uses. Some people swear that drinking a cup of this delightful brew daily has eradicated their age spots completely over a period of time. It tastes so good that it can't hurt to try it. Dandelion is chock full of vitamins purported to give the skin a youthful glow, plus it contains hepatic, aperient, and detoxifying properties.

**1 CUP WATER**

**2 TEASPOONS DANDELION ROOTS, LEAVES, OR FLOWERS**

Bring water to a boil, then add herbs. Remove from heat, cover, and steep for six minutes. Strain and, if desired, add sweetener of choice. Compost or discard herbs.

## ESSENTIAL OIL: *Essential Oil Cream*

Frankincense is a resin that is well known for its lightening properties. Using this in your daily face cream will not only help your skin, age spots, and wrinkles, it will also smell heavenly.

**10 DROPS FRANKINCENSE**

**1 OUNCE LOTION (USE YOUR FAVORITE)**

Mix the essential oils with your face cream. Be sure to stir before each usage, as the oils tend to rise to the top. Apply to face as usual, ensuring that you cover the age spots well with the cream. Do not get into your eyes. Keep in a jar with a tight-fitting lid for up to two months.

## HOME REMEDY: *Age Spot Tips*

There are so many home remedies that a lot of people swear by and have used for years. Try incorporating a few of these into your daily life for reducing and preventing age spots.

- Vitamins C and E are good for the skin and for fighting the harmful effects of the sun.

- Rubs: castor oil, aloe vera, lemon, apple cider vinegar, buttermilk, fresh lemon juice, or onion. Choose one of these and rub it on your age spots daily to get the lightening of your skin that you desire.

- Wear a hat when you go outside, use sunscreen daily, and stay in the shade when possible.

• • • •

# ALLERGIES (SEASONAL)

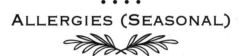

For thousands of years, people have used several of the recipes below for their many decongesting therapeutic properties. Allergies can be caused by various substances that are present in the air that we breathe. They zap our energy, make it difficult for us to concentrate, and make sleep and easy breathing a distant memory. These recipes are proven allergy fighters and can help you to get back to your normal, energetic, happy self.

## AYURVEDA: *Allergy Infusion*

My favorite herb in the entire universe is thyme. This herb is used in almost every culture to cut congestion, clear the sinuses, relieve sore throats, unstop breathing passages, and bring about respiratory relief.

**4 TEASPOONS THYME LEAVES**

**1 CUP WATER**

Steep the leafy parts of fresh or dried thyme in a cup of boiling water for ten minutes. Strain and, if desired, add sweetener of choice or lemon. Compost or discard herbs. Sip throughout the day by the teaspoonful when you have congestion or headaches.

## HERB: *Double Mint Herbal Tea*

Mints are often overlooked as the great healers that they are. Mints contain so many healing properties that it is hard to list them all. A few of the properties that work well when you have seasonal allergies are the expectorant, analgesic, anti-inflammatory, antiphlogistic, antispasmodic, decongestant, and sudorific components. This tea will bring you instantaneous relief when your sinuses and lungs are full of crud.

**1 CUP WATER**

**1 TEASPOON PEPPERMINT**

**1 TEASPOON SPEARMINT**

Bring water to a boil, then add herbs. Remove from heat, cover, and steep for six minutes. Strain and, if desired, add sweetener of choice or lemon. Compost or discard herbs.

## ESSENTIAL OIL: *Allergy Diffuser*

These two essential oils will work magic in the air. They are full of decongestant, analgesic, anti-inflammatory, and expectorant healing properties. As an added bonus, they will make your home smell great!

**4 DROPS LEMONGRASS OIL**

**4 DROPS LAVENDER OIL**

**WATER**

Add oils and water to diffuser and run as desired.

## HOME REMEDY: *Seasonal Fruit Salad*

This is my go-to salad every spring and fall when I get allergies the most. I try to eat this salad at least every week. It is so loaded with compounds in each bite that are full of healthy properties such as antidepressant, decongestant, cephalic, magnesium, immune boosting, antimicrobial, anti-infective, anti-inflammatory, antiviral, bactericidal, expectorant, quercetin, and tonic agents. Your allergies don't stand a chance against this home remedy that tastes so good!

1 APPLE, CORED AND DICED

⅛ CUP WALNUTS, CHOPPED

¼ RED ONION, DICED

1 CUP FRESH LETTUCE BLEND

2 TABLESPOONS FRESH OR DRIED THYME LEAVES

2 TABLESPOONS HONEY

1 TEASPOON LEMON JUICE

Mix the first four ingredients together. In a smaller bowl, mix the last three ingredients together as a dressing. Stir into your salad and enjoy. If you eat this salad along with drinking a cup of orange juice, you will boost your vitamin C intake and take charge of those sinuses. Store remainder, tightly covered, in refrigerator for up to twenty-four hours.

• • • •

# ANXIETY

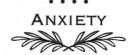

Anxiety is an unnatural feeling caused by stress, fear, or an often undetermined cause. Someone suffering from anxiety does not have inner peace or grounding due to chronic stress from worry, fear, or a chemical imbalance. Therapy and medical intervention should be sought if anxiety is affecting serious areas of your life. There are medications on the market today that use chemicals to produce feelings of calm and ease in the mind, but these sometimes come with even more harmful side effects. Many people have turned to more natural, chemical-free remedies to alleviate fears. These recipes have been handed down for generations to help combat those long worrisome nights and social anxiety dilemmas we all face from time to time.

## AYURVEDA: *Anti-Anxiety Treatments*

Ayurvedics believe in the holistic approach to healing someone suffering from anxiety. This involves the body, mind, diet, thoughts, and spirit. Working on all of these areas will not only decrease your anxiety, but also have you living a happier, more fulfilling lifestyle. Try one or more of the following techniques to curb anxiety, fear, and paranoia:

- Try alternate nostril breathing. Sit comfortably, bring the right thumb up, and place it on the right side of your right nostril, palm facing the mouth, and close the nostril. Close the eyes and breathe deeply through the left nostril five times. Repeat entire sequence on left side.

- Decrease the vata dosha in yourself. Vata is out of balance in people with a high level of anxiety. The vata diet consists of heavy, grounding foods. This adds substance to the soul and body, and thoughts will not run rampant like the air. Eat several small meals a day and avoid getting full. Included in this diet are brown rice, herbal teas, a small amount of wine, carrots, nuts, radishes, potatoes, dairy, tomatoes, corn, ghee (grass-fed if available), and peas. Avoid light, airy foods such as cauliflower, sugar, broccoli, cucumber, asparagus, lettuce, and onions.

- Surround yourself with grounding colors: oranges, greens, browns, and deep, earthy colors. These colors work like magic to settle your nerves and bring peace and relaxation. Stay away from the colors blue and white.

- Hold and look at deep-hued gems such as amethyst, citrine, amber, and crystals. They will ground you and keep your mind from going wild with fear, paranoia, and anxiety. Place one of the gems on the head of your bed and sleep well as you absorb the stone's grounding properties.

- Nature is the best source of peaceful feelings. Take a little walk. Sit on a blanket and meditate while thinking of a tree or flower. Notice the sky, the birds, and the insects working on the ground. We are tiny and insignificant compared to the order of nature. Our fears and worries only hinder our journey on this wonderful path. Enjoy your time outdoors and banish all negative thoughts as soon as they arise. You can train your brain.

- Listen to deep, soothing music. Stay away from hard, pulsing music, which will increase your heart rate and not let your brain settle into a peaceful rhythm. Try listening to some Zen music or Gregorian chants to calm you and leave you feeling peaceful and relaxed.

- Calming the mind is the number one concern for overly anxious people. Meditation teaches us how to direct our thoughts and enjoy our surroundings. Start off meditating five to ten minutes each day. Concentrate on your breathing, and try to banish any negative thoughts. You can train your brain.

- Try prayers of gratitude. I use mala beads to get in tune with my spiritual side. I touch each bead as I say a prayer of thanks for the gifts I have received, and I also say a prayer of thanks for those gifts I have not yet received... but I will! If you name what you want or need and know what you want, be grateful for that thing before you get it; it is already yours. Anxiety has been shown clinically to be reduced dramatically by prayer and meditation.

## HERB: *Anti-Anxiety Herbal Tea*

This recipe is thousands of years old and is proven to be an effective calming agent with its anti-anxiety and sedative properties. This is the first recipe that comes to mind when I know someone is having a hard time with anxiety.

**1 CUP WATER**

**2 TEASPOONS CHAMOMILE FLOWERS**

Bring water to a boil, then add herbs. Remove from heat, cover, and steep for six to eight minutes. Strain and, if desired, add sweetener of choice. Compost or discard herbs.

## ESSENTIAL OIL: *Anti-Anxiety Powder*

Sprinkling this powder under your sheets and pillow cases does wonders for calming the mind and soothing the soul. The antidepressant, anti-anxiety, nervine, and sedative properties work together to quiet those racing thoughts and allay your fears.

**8 DROPS CLARY SAGE OIL**

**3 DROPS YLANG-YLANG OIL**

**3 DROPS ROSE OIL**

**4 DROPS VITAMIN E OIL**

**¼ CUP CORNSTARCH**

Place the ingredients into a mason jar, stirring well. Carefully poke holes into the lid and use this as a shaker to dispense the ingredients into pillowcases or under sheets as needed. You can get a piece of plastic wrap and place it over the jar and under the lid to keep powder from spilling out when not in use. Label and store in a cool, dark, dry area for up to three months.

**HOME REMEDY:** *Spicy Anti-Anxiety Drink*

The calming ingredients in this blend will have you feeling wonderful very quickly. Nutmeg is a stimulating, carminative, digestive spice, and the honey has anti-anxiety properties. The vitamins and minerals in this drink will give you energy and help you to focus on other issues and to not worry needlessly about every minor thing.

> 1 CUP ORANGE JUICE
>
> 1 TABLESPOON HONEY
>
> 1 TEASPOON NUTMEG

Mix the ingredients together in a glass and drink slowly, stirring often.

• • • •

# ARTHRITIS

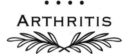

There is a huge variety in the types of arthritis, but one thing they all have in common is pain! Arthritis sufferers have explored so many types of remedies to bring relief to their aching bones and joints. Many of these recipes have proved to work well, and that's why they have been around for hundreds and even thousands of years. Experiment with these recipes, hints, and tips from all over the world to bring relief to your pain and mobility.

**AYURVEDA:** *Arthritis Approach*

Ayurveda attributes arthritis to poor digestion. Using dietary improvements and holistic treatments that improve the digestive tract are also thought to heal arthritis. Ayurveda teaches us to treat our arthritis according to our doshas, either vata, pitta, or kapha.

- A more general type of treatment for all dosha types includes detoxification for five to fourteen days. You can do this by eating mainly light vegetables, juicing, and using herbs and herbal teas in your diet.

- Colonic cleanses are also recommended as a way to assist in detoxifying the body.

- Yoga poses such as tree, forward bend, and waist twists are all helpful in working out the pain of arthritis. These poses are detoxifying, and twists are especially helpful in ridding the body of toxins. Do not strain, but gently go into some stretching poses, and every day you will find yourself in positions that you never thought you would achieve.

- All dosha types should also include ginger, garlic, turmeric, and cayenne pepper in the diet as often as possible as they contain powerful detoxifying, pain relieving, and antiarthritic components.

- You can also utilize alternating heat and ice packs placed on the sore joints and muscles. This age-old technique is good for quick temporary pain relief.

HERB: *Herbal Arthritis Balm*

This rub includes herbs that are specifically targeted to heal and soothe painful and inflamed joints and muscles. These herbs include such healing elements as analgesic, anesthetic, anti-inflammatory, antispasmodic, and febrifuge properties.

1 CUP SESAME OIL

¼ CUP WILLOW BARK

¼ CUP PEPPERMINT LEAVES

1 OUNCE BEESWAX PELLETS

5 DROPS VITAMIN E OIL

Put sesame oil in a glass or stainless-steel pan and heat on stovetop or in oven on very low heat. Add crushed willow bark and peppermint leaves to the oil and stir. Lower heat to warm and heat for an hour, stirring occasionally.

Strain through cheesecloth into jar. Compost or discard herbs. Add beeswax and vitamin E oil and stir until wax is dissolved. Pour into desired container. Label and date the container. Cool mixture completely before using. Rub mixture on the sore and painful joints. Keep away from sensitive areas such as genitals, eyes, inner ears, mouth, mucus membranes, or open wounds. You may use a bandage or gauze to cover as mixture can stain furniture and clothing. Store remainder in a cool, dark area for up to one year.

## ESSENTIAL OIL: *Arthritis Oil Bath*

When your bones hurt and feel stiff and painful, this bath will relax and melt you into such a pain-free condition that you won't want to get out. The agents at work in these essential oils include analgesic, antispasmodic, anti-inflammatory, nervine, sedative, and tranquilizing therapeutic properties.

> 4 DROPS MARJORAM OIL
>
> 4 DROPS SAGE OIL
>
> 6 DROPS VETIVER OIL
>
> 1 TABLESPOON SESAME OIL
>
> 1 TABLESPOON MILK (OPTIONAL)

As you fill the tub with water, pour the essential oils and sesame oil into the running water. Run a warm bath. Water that is too hot will cause the essential oils to dissipate. If you add milk to the water, it will prevent the oil from floating on top of the water and sticking to your skin. Soak for as long as you are comfortable.

## HOME REMEDY: *Yoga Forward Elbow Bend*

This simple yogic exercise is the best arthritic back pain reliever I have ever used. I do this pose several times daily for instant relief.

Stand straight and tall. Slowly bend at the waist as if touching your toes. Hang in this position for five breaths. Grab opposite elbows with your hand while in a hanging position. Slowly turn your head and neck from side to side while continuing to hold your elbows and breathe deeply. Imagine that all of your pain is flowing through your spine and out through the top of your head. You will feel instant back relief from this pose.

# ATHLETE'S FOOT

Athlete's foot is a painful, itchy, ugly condition. It usually attacks people who tend to wear socks and shoes in all weather and people who sweat in their feet. Many dietary conditions can make fungus grow on the feet, and sugar is the primary culprit in these cases. There are numerous reasons why certain lifestyles cause people to get athlete's foot. Many recipes have evolved throughout the ages to rid one of this fungal infection.

## AYURVEDA: *Cinnamon Foot Bath*

Ayurvedic practitioners use cinnamon to relieve athlete's foot issues. The cinnamon has fungal-fighting properties and also helps to end itching.

**6–9 CINNAMON STICKS**

**4 CUPS WATER**

Break up the sticks into two-inch pieces. Put into a pan with water and simmer on stove for five to seven minutes. Cover and steep for thirty to sixty minutes. Once mixture cools to a warm temperature, strain and pour into a flat-bottomed bowl or pan. Use liquid as a foot bath and soak feet in mixture until temperature is no longer comfortable, around twenty minutes. Dry feet very well, especially between the toes. Discard remainder.

## HERB: *Tea Foot Bath*

This bath feels so good and relaxing to itchy, tired feet. Tea has natural tannins and astringents that will help to heal your feet while soothing them at the same time. These tea herbs have analgesic, vulnerary, anti-inflammatory, antibiotic, antiseptic, antiviral, disinfectant, antimicrobial, deodorant, and detoxifying healing properties.

**3 CUPS WATER**

**2 TEASPOONS CALENDULA FLOWERS**

**2 TEASPOONS LAVENDER FLOWERS**

**2 TEASPOONS THYME LEAVES**

Bring water to a boil. Place herbs in a piece of cheesecloth for easy disposal. Pour water over the teabag in a large container with a flat bottom. Cover and let sit for ten to fifteen minutes. When mixture has cooled slightly, place your feet into the container of tea and sit for ten to twenty minutes or until the water is no longer comfortable. Dry feet very well after you are done, and you may sprinkle your feet with a light dusting of cornstarch.

## ESSENTIAL OIL: *Oil Fungus Killer*

These essential oils have worked for centuries in healing athlete's foot and other fungal ailments. The components of this blend include astringent, detoxifying, anti-inflammatory, antifungal, antimicrobial, anti-infective, vermifuge, and anti-parasitic healing properties. Use this recipe often and continue to use it daily for at least a week after all signs of fungal attack have dissipated.

- **4 DROPS PEPPERMINT OIL**
- **2 DROPS LEMON OIL**
- **2 DROPS LEMONGRASS OIL**
- **2 DROPS PATCHOULI OIL**
- **3 DROPS VITAMIN E OIL**
- **1 TABLESPOON CARRIER OIL (SUCH AS JOJOBA, SESAME, GRAPESEED, OR YOUR PREFERENCE)**

Mix the ingredients in a small glass container and apply lightly to the area in and around your toes and feet. Your feet will be slippery when you walk, so rest with feet up for ten minutes to allow most of the oils to be absorbed into your skin. Then slip on some slippers before walking to keep the oils from staining floor and carpet, and to keep you from sliding and falling. Keep essential oil mixture away from open wounds, mucus membranes, genitals, eyes, and sensitive areas. Repeat application as needed, usually two to three times daily. Store unused portion in a glass jar with a tight-fitting lid, label it, and keep it in a cool, dark area for up to six months.

## HOME REMEDY: *Athlete's Foot Home Remedies*

- Only wear clean white cotton socks. Change them often and don't wear them once they get wet.

- Dry feet and toes well after bath and anytime they get wet.

- Make a paste out of one teaspoon baking soda and a half teaspoon water. Apply to feet for instant relief of itching. Rinse your feet and dry them well once the paste has dried to a crust.

- Make a footbath of five cups water and one-third cup lemon juice. Soak your feet and dry well when done.

• • • •

# BACK PAIN

Genetics play a large part in many cases of back pain, as does overexertion, diet, and exercise. People have been trying to bring relief to their aching backs since before the pyramids were built in Egypt. These are some of the remedies that have brought much-needed relief to countless numbers of people who suffer from chronic back pain.

## AYURVEDA: *Lower Back Ointment*

The lower back tends to hurt more as we age. Whether due to arthritis, a slipped disc, or a pulled muscle, this age-old Ayurvedic treatment can relieve the pain and bring comfort. These ingredients have many therapeutic properties, including antiarthritic, detoxifier, antispasmodic, anti-inflammatory, tonic, and vulnerary components.

### ¼ CUP COCONUT OIL

### 4 GARLIC CLOVES, MINCED

Heat coconut oil in a small pan until almost hot. Briskly heat the minced garlic in the coconut oil until garlic is tender, about one minute. Cool until warm. Strain and discard garlic. Rub mixture on the muscles of the back until it is absorbed into the skin. Repeat morning and night or when back pain is most severe. Keep remainder in a jar with a tight-fitting lid in a cool area for up to three days.

## HERB: *Wonder Back Salve*

This salve has enough herbal power to relieve that chronic pain and let you have a good day or a good night's sleep. Easy to prepare, it makes enough to last for a long time. These herbs contain analgesic, antidepressant, antispasmodic, anti-inflammatory, anesthetic, and sedative healing properties.

½ CUP WHITE WILLOW BARK

½ CUP ST. JOHN'S WORT

½ CUP FENNEL

½ CUP BIRCH BARK

1 TABLESPOON GROUND TURMERIC

1 TEASPOON GRATED GINGER

2 CUPS CARRIER OIL (SUCH AS JOJOBA, SESAME, GRAPESEED, OR YOUR PREFERENCE)

5 DROPS VITAMIN E OIL

1–2 OUNCES BEESWAX, GRATED

Pack the herbs into carrier oil and cook on extremely low heat for 1½ hours. Strain through cheesecloth, being careful to not burn yourself, and discard the herbs. Add vitamin E to the oil, then add between one and two ounces of beeswax, depending on whether you like it thicker or thinner. Stir until beeswax is melted. Pour into a jar and label. Cool before applying to skin. Apply to back pain area by rubbing into the skin. Store remainder in a cool, dark area for up to six months. This mixture will stain clothing or furniture, so you may want to cover the area with gauze or wear an old T-shirt.

## ESSENTIAL OIL: *Pain Elimination Bath Salts*

This recipe has such a good outcome not only for your aching back, but also for your overall spirit. These essential oils have analgesic, anti-neuralgic, antispasmodic, tonic, and anti-inflammatory healing properties.

2 TABLESPOONS CARRIER OIL (SUCH AS JOJOBA, SESAME, GRAPESEED, OR YOUR PREFERENCE)

5 DROPS CAJEPUT OIL

5 DROPS MYRRH OIL

5 DROPS BASIL OIL

**3 CUPS SALT (PINK HIMALAYAN, SEA, EPSOM, OR YOUR PREFERENCE)**

**1 TABLESPOON MILK (OPTIONAL)**

Add the oils to the salt. Stir until well blended. Cover tightly. Leave mixture in a dark area for twenty-four hours, then stir mixture again. Run the bathwater, but not so hot as to ruin the oils. Add a half cup bath salt mixture to bathwater. If you add milk to the water, it will prevent the oil from floating on top of the water and sticking to your skin. Store remainder in a container with a tight-fitting lid in a cool, dark area for up to three months. These jars make attractive, inexpensive, and healing gifts!

**HOME REMEDY:** *Back Pain Tips*

- Walk outside and enjoy nature. It's amazing how peaceful and mind-clearing a walk in the woods can be. Walking also strengthens our core muscles, which, in turn, support our backs.

- Music really can calm the savage beast. Music affects every part of our body, mind, and soul. Listen to music that you love. You will feel relaxed and so much calmer, reducing your stress and thereby releasing the muscles of your back.

- Try to get 7–8 hours of sleep every night. Even people who don't suffer from back pain complain of stiff muscles and joints when they don't get enough sleep.

- Drink some herbal tea. The healing properties in herbs, along with the slow ritual of drinking a hot cup of tea, can calm and relax your muscles like nothing else.

- Alternate ice packs followed by heat packs on your back. The anti-inflammatory effects of ice and the blood-pumping effects of the heat can have profound adjustments where you need them most.

- No caffeine, lots of veggies, no alcohol, and no sugar can go a long way in helping you get in shape and ending inflammation.

- Do any type of exercise you wish, but abdominal exercises will help you to better support your back. Strengthening your core is the key. Yoga, walking, stretching, and swimming can all help you improve your back and get you on the road to a rapid recovery.

• • • •

# BAD BREATH (HALITOSIS)

Bad breath, or halitosis, can leave a lasting impression on people. Oral hygiene is at the top of the list when it comes to reasons for halitosis, but there can be other mitigating factors such as illness, food, and sleep. These recipes have been around forever—because they work.

## AYURVEDA: *Halitosis Spoon*

In Ayurveda curing bad breath is easy and delicious. These healing properties don't just cover up the smell of bad breath, they go to work with vigor in treating and healing the causes.

¼ TEASPOON FRESH LEMON JUICE

⅛ TEASPOON GRATED GINGER

1 TABLESPOON HONEY

Combine the ingredients into a large spoon and swallow. Repeat daily until halitosis is no longer an issue.

## HERB: *Clean Mouth Herbal Tea*

This refreshing tea has such a good flavor that you won't notice it is doing its job as an antibacterial, antimicrobial, and anti-inflammatory warrior to the germs in your mouth that breed halitosis.

1 CUP WATER

1 TEASPOON PEPPERMINT LEAVES

1 TEASPOON SPEARMINT LEAVES

Bring water to a boil, then add herbs. Remove from heat, cover, and steep for six to eight minutes. Strain and, if desired, add sweetener of choice. Compost or discard herbs.

## ESSENTIAL OIL: *Halitosis Gargle*

This refreshing drink has antibacterial and antimicrobial properties that will kill those germs and leave your mouth feeling fresh and tingly.

1 CUP WATER

1 TEASPOON BAKING SODA

2 DROPS PEPPERMINT OIL

Combine all ingredients into a glass. Put a small amount into your mouth and rapidly swish around. Spit it all out when done; do not swallow. Repeat until mouth feels clean. Store remainder in a jar with a tight-fitting lid in a cool, dark area for up to twenty-four hours.

## HOME REMEDY: *Good Breath Chew*

There are so many different herbs used all over the world that people chew to put an end to their bad breath. In many countries you can't just run to the store and get a bottle of mouthwash. People simply use what grows around them to make their breath sweet and clean. This recipe is simple, easy, and yummy: grab a sprig or some seeds and chew! The following herbs and seeds will provide you with fresh-smelling breath for hours: fennel seed, basil leaves, parsley leaves, mint leaves, lemon thyme leaves, and cloves.

· · · ·

# BED WETTING (ENURESIS)

Bed wetting, or enuresis, affects numerous people, usually young boys, and it often ends right before puberty. When adults have enuresis, it is sometimes due to an underlying illness or possibly inebriation or drugs. A diagnosis should be sought in the event that an adult has recurring issues with urinating while sleeping. Some of the recipes and tips below can help with occasional bouts of enuresis.

## AYURVEDA: *Enuresis Treatment*

Ayurvedic treatments for bedwetting are safe and easy. There are two main treatments that are used in Ayurveda: one of them involves essential oils, and the other is this drink. Turmeric is an anti-inflammatory and an immune stimulant. Honey has healing benefits and is also an anti-inflammatory.

¼ TEASPOON TURMERIC

1 TEASPOON HONEY

1 GLASS MILK OR WATER

Combine ingredients together and mix with milk or water. Drink every day. Remainder may be refrigerated for up to twenty-four hours.

## HERB: *Herbal Enuresis Tincture*

The known diuretic and calming properties of these herbs have been used forever to curb enuresis. Take this tincture an hour before bed each night and enjoy an uninterrupted night of sleep.

2 TABLESPOONS HORSETAIL

2 TABLESPOONS PLANTAIN LEAVES

2 TABLESPOONS CHAMOMILE FLOWERS

2 TABLESPOONS LEMON BALM LEAVES

1 ½ CUPS VEGETABLE GLYCERIN OR VODKA

Place herbs in a pint jar until it's half full with dried herbs or two-thirds full with fresh herbs, and cover with a high proof vodka (for adults) or vegetable glycerin (for children), about an inch from the top of the jar. Cover tightly and place in a cool, dark location. Shake vigorously every day for two weeks, then let it set without shaking for one month. Strain, bottle, and label, adding the date you decanted it (strained the herbs). Use a half to one dropperful in tea, water, or other liquid. If kept in a cool, dark place, tinctures will last several years if made with alcohol or one year for vegetable glycerin.

## ESSENTIAL OIL: *Enuresis Oil Rub*

These oils are known for their calming properties and are thought to end bladder spasms and lead to a peaceful night's sleep without any "accidents."

**4 DROPS CHAMOMILE OIL**

**4 DROPS LAVENDER OIL**

**3 DROPS VITAMIN E OIL**

**1 TABLESPOON CARRIER OIL (SUCH AS JOJOBA, SESAME, GRAPESEED, OR YOUR PREFERENCE)**

Mix the ingredients in a small glass container and apply lightly to the area desired, such as abdomen, lower back, or soles of feet. Keep essential oil mixture away from open wounds, mucus membranes, genitals, eyes, and sensitive areas. Repeat application as needed, usually once nightly. Store unused portion in a glass jar with a tight-fitting lid in a cool, dark area for up to six months.

## HOME REMEDY: *Enuresis Remedy*

It has been a remedy for years to use walnuts, fennel seeds, and raisins for bed-wetting. The healing elements of these natural foods are reported to stop bed-wetting and help a person wake when the need arises to urinate.

**1 TEASPOON HONEY**

**1 TABLESPOON WALNUTS, CHOPPED**

**1 TEASPOON RAISINS, CHOPPED**

**½ TEASPOON FENNEL SEEDS**

Mix the ingredients together and eat on salad, on a piece of toast, or alone. It tastes like a dessert but works wonders on healing and supporting the urinary tract.

• • • •

# BIPOLAR DISORDER

Bipolar disorder is a mental illness that is marked by a period of mania followed by a period of depression. Heredity has been shown to be a major factor in having bipolar disorder. Learning to balance oneself mentally, physically, and spiritually may be the best defense we have in combating this disorder. Bipolar disorder is a lifelong illness that requires constant monitoring. A good support system with friends and family can often be the biggest weapon of all in battling this illness. Many drugs and therapies are available today to assist people with managing their mood swings. It's important to seek treatment and to consult with your doctor about using essential oils, home remedies, Ayurveda, or herbs combined with prescribed medications as sometimes these treatments render the medications useless or can even be dangerous.

## AYURVEDA: *Remedies for Bipolar Disorder*

An imbalance of the doshas is thought to be responsible for bipolar disorder. However, anyone can benefit from incorporating a few of these grounding practices in their lives. Balancing the moods is the number one goal in controlling bipolar disorder.

- Surround yourself with tones of yellow, green, brown, gold, violet, and earth for balancing and grounding.

- Warm, heavy foods will ground and calm a person with bipolar disorder. Try carrots, potatoes, warm vegetables, baked meats, and heavy foods. Stay away from light, airy foods such as raw vegetables, fruits, and sugar.

- Slow yoga poses and movements will help to calm and center you. Developing a daily practice adds a sense of routine, which is very important for stabilizing moods. Doing yoga, meditation, praying, or exercise outside in the midst of nature is really calming and centering.

- Sit cross-legged and close your eyes. Observe but don't react to your thoughts and concentrate on your breathing. Start out with five minutes a day and increase to twenty minutes per day over time. Learning how to meditate is probably the single most important healing activity for someone with bipolar disorder and can bring about miraculous results.

- Be grateful daily for the things you have, and, more importantly, be grateful for those things that you have yet to receive. If you give thanks for the future you desire, show belief that you will achieve your dreams, and thank your provider for allowing you to have what you do not yet have, it will be yours.

## HERB: *Tea for Bipolar Disorder*

This tea has a leveling effect on the moods, making one calm and content. These herbs are full of tranquilizing and mood-stabilizing properties.

> 1 CUP WATER
>
> 1 TEASPOON BEE BALM LEAVES
>
> 1 TEASPOON GINSENG, GRATED

Bring water to a boil, then add herbs. Remove from heat, cover, and steep for six to eight minutes. Strain and, if desired, add sweetener of choice. Compost or discard herbs.

## ESSENTIAL OIL: *Mood Spray*

Essential oils have been shown to calm a person down from a manic high or lift them up from a bout of depression to feeling Zen. This recipe will help with grounding, calming, and stabilizing a person's moods and bringing them to the place that they desire to be. These oils contain antidepressant, stimulant, tonic, restorative, and calming properties. This blend brings all of the doshas into balance and will help you to achieve that "normal" mood level you desire.

> 10 DROPS ROSE OIL
>
> 10 DROPS FRANKINCENSE OIL
>
> 5 DROPS BASIL OIL
>
> 1 TEASPOON WITCH HAZEL
>
> 2 OUNCES WATER

Combine the ingredients into a spray bottle and shake well. Lightly spray the area desired, such as body, home, or car, and allow to air-dry. Do not spray into eyes, genitals, open wounds, or mucus membranes. Shake well before each use. Store in a cool, dark area for up to three months.

## HOME REMEDY: *Bipolar Home Massage Oil*

Getting a massage can be such a calming and almost a spiritual experience for most people. A person with bipolar disorder can receive numerous benefits from getting this rubdown. The oils in this rub balance out the mind, body and soul with their calming and antidepressant properties.

5 DROPS CLARY SAGE OIL

3 DROPS LEMON BALM (MELISSA) OIL

3 DROPS ROSE OIL

4 DROPS VITAMIN E OIL

1 OUNCE CARRIER OIL (SUCH AS JOJOBA, SESAME, GRAPESEED, OR YOUR PREFERENCE)

Mix the ingredients in a small glass container and massage lightly to the area desired, such as pressure points, neck, soles of feet, temples, back and chest. Keep essential oil mixture away from open wounds, mucus membranes, genitals, eyes and sensitive areas. Repeat application as needed, usually two times daily. Store unused portion in a glass jar with a tight-fitting lid in a cool, dark area for up to six months.

• • • •

# BLOATING

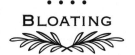

Bloating is that uncomfortable feeling in your abdominal area that leaves you feeling tired and sluggish. Due to menstruation, overeating, or certain medications and illnesses, our stomachs and intestines can trap pockets of air and gasses that swell up and make our lives miserable … not to mention our jeans won't fit! Try a few of these remedies from around the world to put an end to that bloated feeling.

## AYURVEDA: *Digestive Seed Tea*

In Ayurveda it's all about what you put in your body and how your body reacts. This infusion is used to reduce bloating and gas.

- 1 TEASPOON CARDAMOM SEEDS
- 1 TEASPOON FENNEL SEEDS
- 1 TEASPOON CUMIN SEEDS
- 1 CUP BOILING WATER

Place the seeds into the cup of water. Steep for thirty minutes to one hour. Strain and discard seeds. Reserve the liquid in a jar with a tight-fitting lid. Sip a spoonful of the infusion once every ten to twenty minutes until bloating is reduced. Store remainder in refrigerator for up to three days.

## HERB: *Digestive Tea*

This tea has the herbs needed to reduce bloating fast. Need to put on a tight dress before going out? Drink a cup of this one hour before leaving the house, and you will look slim and sleek.

- 1 CUP WATER
- 1 TEASPOON PEPPERMINT OR SPEARMINT LEAVES
- ½ TEASPOON GRATED GINGER

Bring water to a boil, then add herbs. Remove from heat, cover, and steep for six to eight minutes. Strain and, if desired, add sweetener of choice. Compost or discard herbs.

## ESSENTIAL OIL: *Tummy Firmer*

Essential oils have long been known to reduce bloating and rid the body of gas with their carminative, anti-inflammatory, and antispasmodic therapeutic properties.

- 6 DROPS CHAMOMILE OIL
- 4 DROPS FENNEL OIL
- 4 DROPS ROSE OIL
- 3 DROPS VITAMIN E OIL
- ½ OUNCE CARRIER OIL (SUCH AS JOJOBA, SESAME, GRAPESEED, OR YOUR PREFERENCE)

Mix the ingredients in a small glass container and apply lightly to the area desired, such as abdomen and lower back area. Keep essential oil mixture away from open wounds, mucus membranes, genitals, eyes, and sensitive areas. Repeat application as needed, usually two times daily. Store unused portion in a glass jar with a tight-fitting lid in a cool, dark area for up to six months.

**HOME REMEDY:** *Preventions for Bloating*

- Eat a ½-inch piece of ginger before meals to prevent bloating.
- Drink all beverages at room temperature, especially with meals. Ice and cold drinks can increase bloating.
- Eat warm, soothing meals. No cold meals, especially no raw cruciferous vegetables.
- Avoid cauliflower, nuts, salt, dairy, broccoli, brussels sprouts, potatoes, and other gas-inducing foods.
- Chew fennel or cumin seeds after eating.
- Chew your food well before swallowing.
- Eat slowly.
- Eat small meals in a relaxing environment. Try eating while listening to music, talking with family members, and no TV.
- Do not eat fruit within an hour of eating meals.
- Take probiotics daily to regulate your digestive tract.

• • • •
# BOILS

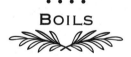

Boils are painful, but relief may be at hand with some of these remedies. It may take some time for boils to come to a head and dissipate, but it is worth the effort to use one of these recipes to get it started. If the boil is infected, produces fever, or is chronic, please seek medical attention immediately.

## AYURVEDA: *Boil Paste*

Turmeric has healing properties such as antifungal, antibacterial, anti-inflammatory, and immune stimulating agents. Apply this paste two to three times daily and cover with a bandage until boil erupts and heals.

**1 TEASPOON TURMERIC**

**1 TEASPOON MILK**

Mix the ingredients together until a thick paste is formed. Smear the paste onto the site. Cover with a bandage, linen, or gauze, as turmeric can stain clothing and furniture. Reapply two to four times daily until wound is healed. Store any remainder in a jar with a tight-fitting lid for up to forty-eight hours.

## HERB: *Echinacea Boil Bandage*

Echinacea has antioxidant, anti-infective, anti-inflammatory, antimicrobial, antiseptic, and cicatrisant properties that will bring the boil to a head and clear it up quickly.

**1 TEASPOON ECHINACEA FLOWERS OR LEAVES**

**½ OUNCE CARRIER OIL (SUCH AS JOJOBA, SESAME, GRAPESEED, OR YOUR PREFERENCE)**

Mix herb with carrier oil and allow to sit overnight. Strain. Apply oil to bandage and place on affected area. Reapply as often as needed.

## ESSENTIAL OIL: *Neem Boil Rub*

Neem is a detoxifier and will clean your wound and help to get rid of the infection. Neem has anti-inflammatory and anti-infective properties.

**5 DROPS NEEM OIL**

**1 TABLESPOON SESAME OIL**

Combine the ingredients in a small bowl. Apply to site several times daily until boil erupts and heals. Store unused portion in a jar with a tight-fitting lid in a cool, dark area for up to three months.

## HOME REMEDY: *Castor Oil Boil Compress*

This is an old home remedy that has been proven to work time and again. Castor oil helps the boil to erupt, thereby opening the way for healing.

**1 TABLESPOON CASTOR OIL**

**BANDAGE OR GAUZE**

Pour the castor oil onto a clean cloth or bandage. Place over the boil. Tape into place and leave on as long as is comfortable. Repeat two to four times daily until boil is healed.

• • • •

# BRONCHITIS

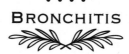

Bronchitis develops when the lungs become inflamed. Treating bronchitis is a very serious matter as it can turn into pneumonia or other life-threatening ailments. It is imperative that you seek medical treatment if symptoms such as fever or infection are present or persist.

## AYURVEDA: *Bronchitis Treatment*

Ayurveda teaches us that bronchitis affects the digestive tract as well as the respiratory organs. Doing yoga, meditation, and other deep-breathing exercises are recommended to help the lungs regain capacity. Completing a cleanse and juicing is also an Ayurvedic approach to ridding the body of bronchitis as well as other toxins. The following drink has antibacterial and anti-inflammatory healing benefits.

**½-INCH PIECE GINGER, DICED**

**1 CUP MILK**

**1 TEASPOON TURMERIC**

Warm the ginger and milk on the stove. Strain to remove ginger pieces. Stir turmeric into the milk and drink a cup at bedtime each night.

## HERB: *Bronchitis Tea*

These herbs are full of decongestant, expectorant, antibacterial, antimicrobial, and analgesic properties to help you get rid of that cough and the chest pain that accompanies bronchitis.

**1 CUP WATER**

**½-INCH GINGER ROOT, DICED**

**¼ TEASPOON CLOVES, CRUSHED**

Bring water to a boil, then add herbs. Remove from heat, cover, and steep for six to ten minutes. Strain and, if desired, add sweetener of choice. Compost or discard herbs.

## ESSENTIAL OIL: *Breathing Well Bath Salts*

This bath salt recipe is so luxurious that you will forget you are sick. The compounds that make up this healing blend are analgesic, antispasmodic, anti-inflammatory, antimicrobial, antiseptic, antiviral, and immunity boosting. These jars make attractive, inexpensive, and healing gifts!

**½ CUP SALT (SUCH AS PINK HIMALAYAN, SEA, EPSOM, OR YOUR PREFERENCE)**

**5 DROPS EUCALYPTUS OIL**

**5 DROPS CEDARWOOD OIL**

**5 DROPS LEMON BALM (MELISSA) OIL**

**1 TABLESPOON CARRIER OIL (SUCH AS JOJOBA, SESAME, GRAPESEED, OR YOUR PREFERENCE)**

**1 TABLESPOON MILK (OPTIONAL)**

Add the oils to the salt. Stir until well blended. Cover tightly. Leave mixture in a dark area for twenty-four hours, then stir again. Run the bathwater, but not so hot as to ruin the oils. Add a half cup of the bath salt mixture to bathwater. If you add milk to the water, it will prevent the oil from floating on top of the water and sticking to your skin. Store remainder in a glass jar with a tight-fitting lid in a cool, dark area for up to three months.

## HOME REMEDY: *Bronchitis Tips*

Home remedies describe simple yet effective treatments or lifestyle changes that can help to rid you of ailments, including mild bronchitis. A medical professional should treat and diagnose chronic bronchitis.

- No smoking or alcohol.
- Drink plenty of room-temperature water to thin the mucus.
- Get lots of rest, and nap when you are tired.
- Alternate hot packs and cold packs on the chest.
- Drink hot herbal teas.
- Take plenty of vitamin C.
- Get fresh air and enjoy nature. Perform mild exercise such as walking outside.
- Take daily Epsom salt baths. The magnesium in the salts is a great healer for most areas of the body.
- Use a humidifier daily.

• • • •

# BURNS

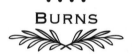

Mild burns can be treated with home remedies, essential oils, herbs, and Ayurvedic treatments. Serious burns require a visit to the emergency room for immediate treatment. Simple burns have been treated with the following recipes for thousands of years.

## AYURVEDA: *Burn Bandage*

In Ayurveda it is common to treat illnesses and injuries as naturally as possible. When someone gets a mild burn, the healing, antiseptic, antibacterial properties of honey can heal burns quickly and painlessly.

¼ TEASPOON HONEY

BANDAGE OR GAUZE

Dab the honey onto a bandage and affix to the site. Leave it on all day and reapply at night. If the burn is very small, you can put a drop of honey directly on the burn without a bandage. Repeat twice daily, as needed.

## HERB: *Plantain-Yarrow Burn Salve*

This is a very effective burn salve as it is loaded with anti-infective, antiseptic, and anti-inflammatory healing properties. Apply as much as three to four times daily.

½ CUP PLANTAIN LEAVES

½ CUP YARROW LEAVES

2 CUPS CARRIER OIL (SUCH AS JOJOBA, SESAME, GRAPESEED, OR YOUR PREFERENCE)

1–2 OUNCES BEESWAX (BEADS OR GRATED)

10 DROPS HEALING ESSENTIAL OILS, SUCH AS LAVENDER OR TEA TREE

½ TEASPOON VITAMIN E OIL

BANDAGE OR GAUZE

Pack the herbs into the carrier oil and cook on low for 1½ hours. Strain through cheesecloth into a glass bowl and add 1 ounce beeswax, stirring until melted. Add essential oils and vitamin E oil and stir. Pour a drop of the mixture onto the counter. Run your finger through the drop after a few seconds of cooling: if it is too thick, add a little oil; if it is too thin, add a little more beeswax. Once you are happy with the consistency, pour into a jar and label. Cool before applying to skin. Apply to desired area by softly rubbing over the skin. Cover lightly with gauze as this mixture will stain clothing and furniture. Reapply every morning and night until burn is healed. Store in a glass jar with a tight-fitting lid in a cool, dark area for up to one year.

## ESSENTIAL OIL: *Burn Drop*

Lavender essential oil has many healing properties to assist in the healing of minor burns and ridding the body of pain instantly. Wait a couple minutes after receiving the burn before applying the oil to the skin.

2–4 DROPS LAVENDER OIL

BANDAGE OR GAUZE

Apply a couple drops of the lavender oil to the mild burn and cover with a bandage. The oil can stain clothing or furniture. Ensure that you are using a safe, 100 percent pure essential oil before placing it on the body, as essential oils can vary greatly from brand to brand.

### HOME REMEDY: *Healing Burn Remedies*

Many remedies work well, and we can make them ourselves very easily for minor burns. More serious burns should always receive medical treatment from a professional. Try a few of these the next time you get a minor scald or heat burn:

- Aloe vera, lavender essential oil, or vitamins C and E rubbed on a burn can speed up healing.
- Food items we have in our cupboards can immediately draw out the heat and the pain: onion juice, cold and wet teabags, vanilla extract, milk, honey, coconut oil, or lemon juice can all work wonders when applied to a minor burn.
- A slice of raw potato laid upon the burn can bring about instant relief.

· · · ·

## CARPAL TUNNEL SYNDROME

Carpal tunnel is a painful experience. Wearing a wrist brace for several months, night and day, is an effective tool in pain relief. Use personal wisdom and seek medical treatment if the pain is chronic. Essential oils, herbs, and Ayurvedic medicine can alleviate pain and reduce swelling at the site of nerve damage or even eliminate the condition altogether.

## AYURVEDA: *Carpal Paste*

This poultice has been known to relieve the intense pain of carpal tunnel. The pain-relieving ingredients contain curcumin properties that bring healing relief.

1 TEASPOON WATER

1 TABLESPOON TURMERIC

BANDAGE OR GAUZE

Mash the water and turmeric together to form a paste. Place directly on the skin or secure into place using a bandage or gauze. Turmeric will stain clothing and furniture. Leave on until no longer comfortable, fifteen minutes to one hour. Reapply each morning and night. Store remainder in a glass jar with a tight-fitting lid in the refrigerator for up to three days.

## HERB: *Carpal Ointment*

Making an ointment out of these therapeutic ingredients can bring fast relief to this painful condition. The healing properties include anti-inflammatory, antispasmodic, antiarthritic, and immune-stimulating agents.

1 OUNCE ARNICA LEAVES

1 OUNCE ST. JOHN'S WORT LEAVES

1 CUP CARRIER OIL (SUCH AS JOJOBA, SESAME, GRAPESEED, OR YOUR PREFERENCE)

6 DROPS VITAMIN E OIL

1 OUNCE BEESWAX, GRATED

Mix the herbs and carrier oil and cook on very, very low heat in the oven for one to three hours or on extremely low heat on the stovetop. Strain, discard herbs, and add vitamin E oil and beeswax; melt and stir well. Pour mixture into a jar. Once cooled, apply as a rub to affected area, such as fingers, wrist, and thumb. You may wish to cover with a bandage, linen, or a light cloth and secure onto the site, as the ointment will stain clothing and furniture. Store remainder in a jar with a tight-fitting lid in a cool, dark area for up to one year.

## ESSENTIAL OIL: *Carpal Tunnel Oil Rub*

There are many healing properties in this oil: anti-inflammatory, analgesic, and anesthetic agents, to name a few of them. This blend feels so good and can help you make it through the night with much-needed relief.

> 1 OUNCE SESAME OIL
>
> 10 DROPS CEDARWOOD OIL
>
> 10 DROPS LAVENDER OIL
>
> 10 DROPS VETIVER OIL
>
> 5 DROPS VITAMIN E OIL

Mix the ingredients in a small glass container and apply lightly to the area desired, such as fingers, thumb, and wrist. Keep essential oil mixture away from open wounds, mucus membranes, genitals, eyes, and sensitive areas. Repeat application as needed, usually two to three times daily. Store unused portion in a glass jar with a tight-fitting lid in a cool, dark area for up to six months.

## HOME REMEDY: *Carpal Tunnel Tips*

These home remedies include common sense and household tips to alleviate the pain of carpal tunnel. Try to incorporate a few of these into your daily living to reduce the inflammation and get on the road to good health.

- Do not eat red meat; stick with lean and white meats. Red meat intensifies inflammation.
- No alcohol, caffeine, or tobacco.
- Take a multivitamin with B6 included.
- Mix 1½ teaspoons flaxseed oil and 1½ teaspoons turmeric together and take by mouth daily to reduce inflammation.
- Alternate between hot and cold compresses applied to the site.
- Wear a splint at all times. Try to not move the affected area, and do not strain or put pressure on it at any time.
- After one month, if carpal tunnel is improving, do a series of wrist and thumb or shoulder stretches two to three times daily.

· · · ·
# CELLULITE

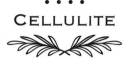

Most people have cellulite. It is a desire by people the world over to even out the skin and have a smoother appearance. Below are some recipes that have been used for generations in various cultures to help smooth that skin out for a sleeker look.

## AYURVEDA: *Cellulite Drink*

This drink is reported to detox the system and get rid of water weight and cellulite. Since it tastes good, give it a try!

> 1 TEASPOON GROUND CAYENNE
>
> 1 TEASPOON GROUND GINGER
>
> ½ TEASPOON LEMON JUICE
>
> 1 GLASS TEPID WATER

Mix the ingredients together and drink this detoxifying, fat-shrinking magic every day for a month or two. You should see the results you want slowly begin to form.

## HERB: *Quick Cellulite Fix*

This is an old remedy that works quickly in a pinch, such as a trip to the beach or wearing that new tight dress. The willow and coffee will work to dehydrate and tighten the skin temporarily.

> 1 CUP HOT COFFEE
>
> 2 TABLESPOONS WHITE WILLOW BARK
>
> LINEN OR CLOTH

Pour the coffee over the herbs and let steep until coffee is mildly warm. Dip a piece of linen or a cloth into the bowl and wring out lightly. Lay this poultice on the desired area of cellulite and let soak in for at least ten to fifteen minutes. Throw away any mixture that is not used.

## ESSENTIAL OIL: *Cellulite Oil Rub*

These essential oils are purported to rid the area of cellulite and detox your saddlebags as well.

**10 DROPS JUNIPER OIL**

**10 DROPS TANGERINE OIL**

**4 DROPS VITAMIN E OIL**

**1 OUNCE ALMOND OIL**

Place the essential oils into a small container. Add the vitamin E and the almond oils. Swirl and use to massage lightly the area desired, especially the saddlebag area (the outer thighs). Keep away from open wounds, eyes, inner ears, mucus membranes, genitals, or sensitive areas. This can be repeated as needed. Store unused portion in a jar with a tight-fitting lid in a cool, dark area for up to one month.

## HOME REMEDY: *Mermaid Cellulite Remedy*

This recipe has been around forever. Kelp and seaweed are known detoxifiers and will help to rid the body of toxins, fats, and waste. Use the products of the ocean to become that mermaid you wish you were.

**½ CUP SEAWEED OR KELP**

**¼ CUP SEA SALT**

**½ CUP EXTRA VIRGIN OLIVE OIL**

Mix the ingredients together and rub on the cellulite area. Massage into the skin using strokes that move upward, toward the heart. Massage area well for five minutes, then rest. After about twenty minutes, wipe off the excess oil. The remainder may be put in a jar with a tight-fitting lid and stored in a cool, dark area for up to two weeks.

· · · ·

## CHAPPED LIPS

We all want smooth, kissable lips, no matter who we are. There are so many ways to keep your lips from wrinkling, cracking, and drying out. Various factors such as allergies, heredity, illness, weather, seasons, and diet can all effect the moisture in our lips. The number one way to keep your lips plump and juicy is to drink water. How simple is that? Below are some ways that people plump up and keep their lips happy from all over the world.

### AYURVEDA: *Lip Healing Tips*

In Ayurveda it is believed that the whole body should be treated to find a cure for a particular body part. Diet, exercise, hydration, and stress can all play a part in how our skin, hair, nails, and lips react and look. These are some tips that Ayurvedic healers believe will have you looking your best.

- Stay hydrated. Drink several glasses of water and sugar-free juice daily.
- Stay away from salt, popcorn, chips, and anything with a high salt content. Eat dandelion greens, beans, fresh veggies, and potatoes.
- Rub sesame oil or ghee on the lips throughout the day. Both will plump and heal the lips.
- The two most powerful weapons against stress buildup are meditation and prayer. Take the time to say prayers or reflect quietly in meditation.

### HERB: *Flower Lip Balm*

There is a saying that you should never put anything on your lips if it doesn't contain calendula! This balm works well as a lip balm. It is healing, plumping, soothing, and has softening agents at work to make your lips the best that they can be.

¼ CUP CARRIER OIL (SUCH AS JOJOBA, SESAME,
   GRAPESEED, OR YOUR PREFERENCE)

¼ CUP CALENDULA FLOWERS

1 OUNCE BEESWAX, SHAVED

7 DROPS VITAMIN E OIL

Combine carrier oil and calendula flowers. Bake in very low oven heat (250–275 degrees) or on a stovetop with very low heat for one hour. Strain and discard herbs. Add beeswax and stir until melted. Cool slightly, then add the vitamin E oil. Drip a couple drops of the mixture onto the counter, wait a few seconds, and run your finger through it. If it is too thick, add more carrier oil. If it is too thin, add more grated beeswax. Once desired consistency is reached, pour into lip balm containers or tins of your choice. Cool. Apply to lips often throughout the day. Store in cool, dark area for up to one year.

## ESSENTIAL OIL: *Oily Chap Balm*

Essential oils work wonders on lips with their healing and therapeutic properties. This little balm is easy to make, and you can put it in a roll-on bottle for easy application and carry it in your purse everywhere you go!

4 DROPS CHAMOMILE OIL

4 DROPS GERANIUM OIL

4 DROPS VITAMIN E OIL

1 TABLESPOON CARRIER OIL (SUCH AS JOJOBA, SESAME,
   GRAPESEED, OR YOUR PREFERENCE)

Combine the ingredients and pour into a roll-on bottle. Apply to lips several times daily. Use within six months.

## HOME REMEDY: *Nutty Lip Licker*

This old remedy is as yummy as it is healthy, but try not to eat it up. Our grandparents didn't know about the chemical components and therapeutic properties of peanut butter and honey; they just knew that this worked in healing dry, cracked lips.

½ TABLESPOON HONEY

½ TABLESPOON SMOOTH PEANUT BUTTER

2 DROPS VITAMIN E OIL

Combine the ingredients with a small whisk or fork in a small bowl. With your finger, apply a light layer of the mixture to your lips. Allow mixture to remain on lips for thirty minutes, then wipe off with a paper towel. Refrigerate remainder for up to three days. Reapply as needed throughout the day for soft, plump, smooth lips.

• • • •

# CIRCULATION (POOR)

Herbs, essential oils, Ayurvedic treatments, and home remedies have been used for thousands of years to help restore blood flow to the limbs. Poor circulation is caused by a myriad of reasons. Your physician can help you to determine the cause of your poor circulation and diagnose if it is caused by a disease.

### AYURVEDA: *Circulation Rice Dish*

In Ayurveda food is often used to transfer healing benefits to the body. This recipe is eaten by people with poor circulation to get the blood flowing with the therapeutic properties in these foods. This recipe will not only help your circulation, but it will work wonders on your entire body. Yummy!

2 TABLESPOONS COCONUT OIL

1 CUP JASMINE OR BASMATI RICE

2 GARLIC CLOVES, MINCED

½-INCH GINGER ROOT, CHOPPED

½ TEASPOON TURMERIC

2 SAFFRON THREADS

In a frying pan, heat the coconut oil, add the rice, and brown lightly over medium heat. When rice begins browning, add minced garlic and ginger and cook for one minute. Add the amount of water recommended on rice package (usually two to three times the amount of the rice). Cook according to package directions. During the last minute of cooking, add turmeric and saffron. Stir, cook for one minute, and enjoy! Store any remainder in the refrigerator in a tightly covered dish for up to three days.

## HERB: *Circulation Tincture*

This tincture has been used for years and has properties to get the blood moving and put an end to poor circulation. This recipe is often used to get the blood circulating in the hands and feet in the winter time.

¼ CUP APPLE CIDER VINEGAR

1 CAYENNE PEPPER, CHOPPED

3 GARLIC CLOVES, MINCED

¼ CUP GINGKO BILOBA

½-INCH GINGER ROOT, MINCED

Mix all the ingredients into a pan. Cook on very low heat for one hour. Strain and discard herbs. Cool the liquid. Take by teaspoonful throughout the day. This is extremely spicy and hot. Drink milk afterwards for a cooling-off effect. Store remainder in the refrigerator for up to two weeks.

## ESSENTIAL OIL: *Blood Flow Massage Oil*

These oils contain circulation-restoring and vasodilator properties. The massage will also heat the blood and get it moving again. You can rub these oils on your legs or have a friend do it for you.

7 DROPS FRANKINCENSE

5 DROPS YLANG-YLANG

5 DROPS LIME

3 DROPS NEROLI

3 DROPS VITAMIN E OIL

1 OUNCE CARRIER OIL (SUCH AS JOJOBA, SESAME, GRAPESEED, OR YOUR PREFERENCE)

Mix ingredients in a glass container and lightly massage the area desired, such as the arms, hands, legs, and feet. Keep essential oil mixture away from open wounds, mucus membranes, genitals, eyes, and sensitive areas. Repeat application as needed. To store unused portion, label a glass jar with a tight-fitting lid and keep in a cool, dark area for up to three months.

### HOME REMEDY: *Circulation Tips*

Here is a list of tips that will help with circulation. These are remedies that have been used forever to help people get that blood pumping. Try one or two of these each day until your circulation improves.

- Use garlic, cayenne, and ginger daily in your diet and eat lots of fibrous fruits and vegetables. Do not use alcohol or tobacco.

- Drink water all day long to stay hydrated. Drink plenty of water before and after meals.

- When you take a shower, begin with hot water, then alternate back and forth between hot and cold water.

- Get a routine of yoga, light exercise, or walking. Try to incorporate some form of exercise into your lifestyle every day.

• • • •

## COLDS

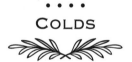

They say we can't come up with a recipe to cure the common cold, but I beg to differ! A cold can be sent on its merry way, quickly, when these remedies are put to use. Get rid of those sniffles, congestion, sneezing, headaches and fatigue when you apply some of these recipes to your daily regimen.

### AYURVEDA: *Steamy Head Clearer*

This timeless Ayurvedic remedy is still commonly used today to drain the sinuses, clear the head, and reduce that mental fogginess associated with having a cold.

½-INCH GINGER ROOT, MINCED

3 CUPS BOILING WATER

Do not use this recipe with children as they can easily scald themselves. Combine ingredients together into a bowl. Be careful not to spill water on yourself. Place a towel over your head and drape it over the bowl, forming a tent over your head. Breathe deeply of the steam that rises from the ginger and water. Once the water cools, place the bowl of water into your bedroom so that you can benefit from the healing vapors released throughout the night. Discard remainder in the morning.

### HERB: *Sniffles Tea*

This tea has decongestant, antispasmodic, anti-inflammatory, and analgesic properties to help you get over that cold. It will even protect you from getting a cold if someone else in the family has one. Make a few cups of this delicious brew and hand it out to everyone in the household during cold and flu season, whether they have a cold or not.

**1 CUP WATER**

**1 TABLESPOON ECHINACEA FLOWERS**

**HONEY**

**JUICE OF ¼ LEMON**

Bring water to a boil, then add herbs. Remove from heat, cover, and steep for six to ten minutes. Strain and add desired amount of honey and lemon. Compost or discard herbs.

### ESSENTIAL OIL: *Breathe Better Diffuser*

Putting these essential oils into the air not only helps you to breathe better, but these properties work to heal and protect your respiratory tract. As an added bonus, your house will smell great!

**4 DROPS EUCALYPTUS OIL**

**4 DROPS SPEARMINT OIL**

**3 DROPS PEPPERMINT OIL**

Add oils and water to diffuser and run as desired.

So many home remedies are effective in eliminating the side effects of the common cold. They work! That's why at least one of these remedies has surely been used on you in your lifetime. Try a couple of these when you have a cold and you are sure to feel better and be on your way to great health.

- Chicken soup has beneficial ingredients that will heal and help you fight a cold. The steam rising from the soup as you eat it is also helpful in clearing out those sinus passages.

- Make sure you dose yourself well with vitamins, drink orange juice, and fight that cold with the healing benefits of vitamin C.

- Take a teaspoon each day of apple cider vinegar, whether in a salad, in a drink, or by itself. Apple cider vinegar is full of therapeutic properties and will kill the cold virus.

- Grate a teaspoon of ginger, mix ⅓ of it with honey and lemon to taste, and take a teaspoonful each day. All three of these ingredients work together like dynamite to kill those cold germs.

- Gargle with a mixture of salt and warm water each morning and evening. Do not swallow the mixture; spit it out. Salt water kills cold germs and will protect you from getting a throat inflammation.

· · · ·

# COLD SORES

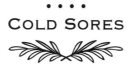

Cold sores (herpes simplex) are ugly, painful, and have no known cure. It seems that people who get cold sores are destined to get them repeatedly. Natural remedies and medications from plants, oils, and other gifts from nature have been used for thousands of years to put an end to these outbreaks.

This recipe is loaded with healing properties such as anti-inflammatory, antiseptic, and antiviral agents. Use this each time you have a cold sore to bring rapid results.

**1 TEASPOON LICORICE ROOT POWDER**

**2 TABLESPOONS PETROLEUM JELLY OR COCONUT OIL**

Combine the ingredients. With fingertips or a cotton swab, apply to cold sore repeatedly throughout the day for two to three days, until cold sore is healed. Discard any remainder after three days.

## HERB: *Echinacea Tea*

Echinacea is a powerful healing herb. These beautiful flowers are renowned for their ability to fight infections and viruses. Drink this tea anytime you have a viral infection like cold sores. These anti-inflammatory and antiviral agents will work quickly to bring an end to those painful sores.

**1 CUP WATER**

**1 TEASPOON ECHINACEA FLOWERS**

Bring water to a boil, then add herbs. Remove from heat, cover, and steep for six to eight minutes. Strain and, if desired, add honey or sweetener of choice. Compost or discard herbs. Keep applying the tea to your lips throughout the day as you drink it and allow the tea to dry onto the cold sore.

## ESSENTIAL OIL: *Healing Lip Balm*

This healing recipe works wonders on the lips. If you wish, you could substitute any number of healing oils with the calendula and spearmint oil, such as grapefruit, peppermint, lemon, or tea tree.

**3–4 TEASPOONS GRAPESEED OIL**

**1 TEASPOON BEESWAX PELLETS**

**4 DROPS VITAMIN E**

**3 DROPS SPEARMINT OIL**

**3 DROPS CALENDULA OIL**

In a glass bowl, heat the grapeseed oil and the beeswax until just melted, using either the stovetop or the microwave. Stir, Pour a drop of the melted oil and wax onto the counter, and after a minute check for consistency. If it is too thin, add more beeswax; if it is too thick, add more grapeseed oil. Add the vitamin E oil and the essential oils to the heated mixture. Whisk lightly, and it will begin hardening immediately. Pour into lipstick containers or small tins or jars. Once cool, apply to cold sore. Reapply throughout the day. Do not apply to mucus membranes, eyes, genitals, or open wounds. Label containers and store in a dark, dry area for up to one year.

HOME REMEDY: *Cold Sore Tips*

These are some tips about various techniques to rid oneself of the herpes simplex virus. Use several of these recipes throughout the day and you will find your cold sore slowly dissipating.

- Make a paste of cornstarch and water and apply often to the lips.
- Dab a little milk onto your cold sore several times a day and let it dry, and it will heal quickly.
- Use a cotton swab soaked in hydrogen peroxide to wet the cold sore three to four times daily until healed.
- Apply witch hazel throughout the day to your cold sore to dry it out and bring relief.
- Eat plenty of salad and berries, which are full of healing properties and will kill the virus causing your cold sore.
- Take an extra dose of vitamins C and E daily until cold sore is gone.

• • • •

## CONCENTRATION

It is so ironic that today I am working on research for concentration. I have been trying to sit at this computer for three hours now. I find myself washing dishes, making vegetable soup, doing yoga, and every other thing under the sun, rather than concentrating on the most important task at hand. Here are a few tips below to get you into that mindset and that desire to accomplish your daily goals. I am about to follow my own advice and get my oils going.

## AYURVEDA: *Focus Meditation*

In Ayurveda practicing focus is the best way to increase the power of concentration. This exercise works well with children and adults. Meditation takes time to understand and feel the benefits. Start out with five minutes twice daily and increase up to twenty minutes or more.

Find a comfortable, quiet area. Outdoors in good weather is the perfect place for meditation. Sit comfortably on the ground or on a pillow. Cross your legs and place your hands, palms up, on your knees. Sit straight and tall. Begin by taking a big breath in and slowly releasing your breath. You can either close your eyes or leave them open and focus on a point of interest. I often just look at a point in the water on the pond. Try to relax and let your mind drift to where it wants to go. If you find yourself getting stressed by your thoughts, take a huge breath in and release, banishing every negative thought. You can chant a word repeatedly in your head or concentrate on your breathing to clear the mind. When you are done, just take a few cleansing breaths and slowly stand. You will feel revitalized, energized, and proud of yourself for focusing and concentrating. Complete this exercise every day until you can meditate with ease and control your own concentration.

## HERB: *Herbal Focus*

This tea helps you focus, concentrate, and increase your ability to retain information. This tea has been used for thousands of years in the Middle and Far East to improve brain function.

> 1 CUP WATER
>
> ½-INCH PIECE GINSENG, PEELED AND DICED
>
> 1 TABLESPOON GINGKO BILOBA

Bring water to a boil, then add herbs. Remove from heat, cover, and steep for eight to ten minutes. Strain and, if desired, add sweetener of choice. Compost or discard herbs.

## ESSENTIAL OIL: *Concentration Roll-On*

These essential oils are known worldwide to support brain function, memory, and concentration. This roll-on recipe is so easy to make, and it will help in school, work, or any task you set your mind to.

**4 DROPS CEDARWOOD OIL**

**4 DROPS VETIVER OIL**

**4 DROPS PEPPERMINT OIL**

**4 DROPS ROSEMARY OIL**

**½ OUNCE SESAME OIL**

**3 DROPS VITAMIN E OIL**

Combine the ingredients and pour into a roller bottle. Roll around the area desired, such as wrist, neck, temples, soles of feet or chest. Do not apply to open wounds, mucus membranes, eyes, or sensitive areas. Shake well before each use. Use daily when concentration is sporadic.

## HOME REMEDY: *Concentration Tips*

We have all tried tricks to get ourselves in the mindset of focusing on a task, concentrating on a conversation, or taking a test. Here are a few of the habits people have used all over the world to give their brain cells a boost.

• There are thousands of types of puzzles. Working on puzzles helps your brain learn to focus and pinpoint exactly what you need to be concentrating on. Puzzles train our brains to stay on track. Puzzles are exercise for the brain.

• Wearing headphones while concentrating on a task will reduce outside noise and keep the interruptions at bay, helping you to focus.

• Drinking plenty of water is not only good for your body, it is also imperative to get the blood flowing properly through your brain.

• Getting the right amount of sleep for yourself is very important. Not getting adequate sleep can cause anyone to be unable to concentrate or focus.

- Make yourself a task list of the things you want to focus on for the next day. When you are ready, begin completing the items on your list, and mark off each task as you complete it. This is the best method I have found to assist me in concentrating on the things I need to get done and to actually finish each project.

- Walking in nature, bike riding, yoga, and numerous other activities will get the blood pumping to your brain. In the same way your body can become stagnant and not operate at full speed without exercise, your brain will respond in kind when it is not fed activities to keep it functioning at its peak.

## • • • •
# CONGESTION

Congestion is an inflammation of the nose, throat, or chest. Being clogged with mucus can cause coughing, hacking, inability to breathe, sore throat, sleepless nights, and a host of other side effects. Various remedies have been used throughout time to heal congestion without harmful chemicals being introduced into an already compromised system.

### AYURVEDA: *Oil Pull*

Ayurveda teaches us that most of a person's germs live in their mouth and teeth. Oil pulling attracts the germs and bacteria to the oil, which you spit out. This is an easy way to detox and rid the body of toxic germs. This practice is thousands of years old. Give it a try the next time you are congested and need a cleansing. It actually does not have a taste and is a much thinner liquid than you may think. Coconut oil is a very powerful antibacterial agent.

Add one tablespoon fractionated coconut oil to a large spoon. Very gently, swish oil between all teeth, over tongue and in all areas of the mouth for ten to fifteen minutes. After you are done, spit all of the oil out of your mouth and into the garbage. Do not swallow the oil. Repeat every morning as needed.

## HERB: *Congestion Herbal Tincture*

This recipe has powerful decongesting therapeutic properties. Make this tincture recipe six weeks before cold and flu season so you will be ready to attack those germs when they arrive.

¼ CUP THYME LEAVES

¼ CUP PEPPERMINT LEAVES

¼ CUP CHAMOMILE LEAVES

¾ CUP VODKA OR VEGETABLE GLYCERIN

Place herbs in a pint jar until it's half full with dried herbs or two-thirds full with fresh herbs, and cover the herbs with a high proof vodka (for adults) or vegetable glycerin (for children), leaving about an inch at the top of the jar. Cover tightly and place in a cool, dark location. Shake vigorously every day for two weeks, then let it set without shaking for one month. Strain, bottle, label, and put the date you decanted it, or strained out the herb. Drink ½–1 dropperful in tea, water, juice, or other liquid two to three times daily until congestion is cleared. If kept in a cool, dark place, tincture made with alcohol will last several years and vegetable glycerin-based tincture will last up to one year.

## ESSENTIAL OIL: *Congestion Wonder Oil*

Placing a drop of this oil on the soles of the feet is one of the most widely used ways to help rid one of congestion. This oil is full of decongestant, antispasmodic, analgesic, anti-inflammatory, antiviral, and antimicrobial therapeutic properties. The uses for this oil blend are limitless. The vitamin E oil acts as a preservative so you can make it ahead and use it when it's needed.

10 DROPS CLOVE OIL

8 DROPS LEMON OIL

8 DROPS TEA TREE OIL

6 DROPS CINNAMON BARK OIL

6 DROPS EUCALYPTUS OIL

4 DROPS ROSEMARY OIL

5 DROPS VITAMIN E OIL

½ OUNCE CARRIER OIL (SUCH AS JOJOBA, SESAME, GRAPESEED, OR YOUR PREFERENCE)

In a small glass container, mix the ingredients together and swirl or stir to evenly disperse the oils. Apply a small amount of the mixture to desired area, such as head, chest, back, or soles of feet, and rub in well. This blend may also be poured into a roll-on bottle. Reapply morning and night. Do not get mixture into eyes, mucus membranes, genitals, or sensitive areas, as the oils are very strong. Store unused portion in a dark glass jar with a tight-fitting lid, label it, and keep it in a cool, dark area for up to six months.

## HOME REMEDY: *Chicken Soup*

Chicken soup really does help with congestion—Grannie knew what she was talking about! All the added benefits from the vitamins and minerals in the vegetables can only help you. The steam from the soup loosens congestion and acts as an expectorant. This recipe is a family favorite and can be whipped up anytime anyone is under the weather from coughing, colds, congestion, or flu.

½ STICK BUTTER

2 CELERY STALKS, DICED

2 GARLIC CLOVES, MINCED

1 ONION, DICED

2 CHICKEN BREASTS, COOKED AND CHOPPED

2 CARROTS, DICED

3 MEDIUM POTATOES, DICED

4 CUPS WATER

1 CAN ROTEL TOMATOES

2 CUPS CHICKEN BROTH

1 TABLESPOON FLOUR

PARSLEY (OPTIONAL)

In a large pot, melt butter over medium burner. Add the celery, garlic, and onion, and cook a couple minutes until translucent. Add the chicken, carrots, potatoes, water, tomatoes, and broth to the pan. Cook over medium heat for thirty minutes. Once potatoes are tender, season with salt and pepper. Five minutes before the soup is ready, whisk the flour with a little water. Add to pan, stirring well, and cook for five minutes until soup is thickened. Top with parsley and serve with crackers.

• • • •

# CONSTIPATION

We all have those periods in our lives when things don't quite come out like they should. Not having your daily bowel movement can lead to crankiness, feeling uncomfortable, and even to serious complications if left untreated for very long periods of time. These recipes have been used worldwide to try to get your colon, intestines, and bowels to perform at their peak.

## AYURVEDA: *Constipation Pull*

Sesame oil is a magnet for toxins and also relieves constipation-causing germs that reside in your mouth. I like to use sesame oil as a pull for many different reasons, including taste, texture, and effectiveness.

**1 TEASPOON SESAME OIL**

Swish a small amount through teeth and mouth for five minutes and then spit out into the garbage. Do not swallow.

## HERB: *Movement Tea*

This tea has been used for generations to relieve the occasional bout of constipation.

**1 CUP WATER**

**1 TEASPOON NETTLE LEAVES**

**1 TEASPOON DANDELION LEAVES**

Bring water to a boil, then add herbs. Remove from heat, cover, and steep for six to eight minutes. Strain and, if desired, add sweetener of choice. Compost or discard herbs. Two to three cups a day will suffice to get movement in the bowels.

## ESSENTIAL OIL: *Oil Pusher*

These essential oils are used for their anti-inflammatory and antispasmodic properties. Used on the abdomen, they can be quite effective in loosening and relieving constipation.

10 DROPS PEPPERMINT OIL

10 DROPS CHAMOMILE OIL

5 DROPS VITAMIN E OIL

½ OUNCE CARRIER OIL (SUCH AS JOJOBA, SESAME,
GRAPESEED, OR YOUR PREFERENCE)

Mix the ingredients in a small glass container and apply lightly to the area desired, such as abdomen and lower back. Wear an old T-shirt to keep the oils from staining your furniture. Keep essential oil mixture away from open wounds, mucus membranes, genitals, eyes, and sensitive areas. Repeat application as needed, usually two to three times daily. Store unused portion in a glass jar with a tight-fitting lid, label it, and keep it in a cool, dark area for up to six months.

## HOME REMEDY: *Old-Timey Smooth Salad*

This is the best-known treatment in many families. We love to treat minor ailments with food when possible, as food is the best medicine known to man (and bad food can be the worst poison). Try this salad to get those bowels in tip-top shape. This salad is tangy, spicy, sweet, and crunchy. These vegetables are full of fiber to help you clean out the colon.

½ TABLESPOON MOLASSES

1 TEASPOON LEMON JUICE

1 HEAD BROCCOLI, CHOPPED (ABOUT 2 CUPS)

1 PLUM, DICED

½ PEAR, DICED

2 TABLESPOONS WALNUTS, CHOPPED

¼ APPLE, DICED

¼ ONION, CHOPPED

½ CUP LETTUCE GREENS, CHOPPED

Whisk together the molasses and lemon juice along with any herbs you may like in your salad (I usually add a clove of minced garlic, lemon thyme, or chives to mine). Combine the rest of the fruits and vegetables together and cover with the salad dressing. This combination of fruits and veggies can really get you running to the bathroom in no time. You may refrigerate remainder for up to three days in a bowl with a tight-fitting lid.

· · · ·
# COUGH

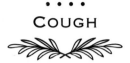

Coughing is a reflex of the lungs and body to rid a person of an unwanted particle in the lungs. There are a host of reasons why a person would begin coughing. A diagnostician can determine what is causing your cough and how to end that cause. Many coughs are caused by viral and bacterial agents. Since time immemorial people have used plants, flowers, food, and other techniques to reduce coughing. If coughing is severe or chronic, seek medical attention.

## AYURVEDA: *Decongestant Spoon*

A spoonful of healing for your lungs and head. These herbs and spices carry a lot of decongesting and sudorific properties to bring you healing and relief.

JUICE OF ½ LEMON (ABOUT 1–2 TEASPOONS)

¼ TEASPOON TURMERIC

1 PINCH BLACK PEPPER

1 PINCH CINNAMON

1 TEASPOON HONEY

Combine ingredients into a large spoon and either mix into a glass of water and drink or swallow the spoonful. I like to mix it with water and drink it all at once. It is strong and will coat your throat with soothing, healing ingredients.

## HERB: *Honey Cough Syrup*

These anti-inflammatory and decongesting herbs will have you feeling better in no time. Taking a teaspoon of this recipe a couple of times a day will have you feeling better and breathing easier quickly. Kids especially love the flavor of this blend.

⅓ CUP THYME LEAVES

1 TABLESPOON GRATED GINGER

½ CUP HONEY

Place herbs in a jar, cover with runny honey (or vegetable glycerin, if you prefer), and put the lid on the jar. Place in a sunny windowsill or a warm spot and leave for two weeks. If the herbs rise above the honey, you will need to press them down into the honey so they won't turn brown. After two weeks, strain and bottle. Take one teaspoon up to three times a day. Store unused portion in a glass jar with a tight-fitting lid, label it, and keep it in a cool, dark area for up to six months.

### ESSENTIAL OIL: *Chest Rub Decongestant*

This is full of therapeutic properties such as sudorific, expectorant, and anti-inflammatory agents. This blend is quite effective at decongesting your lungs and head.

5 DROPS TEA TREE OIL

5 PEPPERMINT OIL

5 DROPS EUCALYPTUS OIL

2 DROPS CLOVE OIL

4 DROPS VITAMIN E OIL

½ OUNCE CARRIER OIL (SUCH AS JOJOBA, SESAME, GRAPESEED, OR YOUR PREFERENCE)

Mix the ingredients in a small glass container and apply lightly to the area desired, such as soles of feet, back, and chest. Protect clothing and furniture from staining by wearing an old T-shirt. Keep essential oil mixture away from open wounds, mucus membranes, genitals, eyes, and sensitive areas. Repeat application as needed, usually two to three times daily. Store unused portion in a glass jar with a tight-fitting lid, label it, and keep it in a cool, dark area for up to six months.

**HOME REMEDY:** *Decongesting Tips*

Here are some simple remedies that have been handed down from one family to another for generations. Try a few of these the next time you start having those coughing fits.

- Take a probiotic according to package directions to keep your immune system in tip-top shape.

- Eat pineapple—it has natural immunity-boosting properties.

- Make a chest rub out of eucalyptus oil, peppermint oil, and coconut oil.

- Drink lots of hot herbal tea.

- Have a steamy shower. The steam will open the breathing passageways.

- Take a spoonful of lemon and honey with a pinch of cayenne pepper.

- Stay hydrated. Thinning out the mucus with water is very effective.

- Let your body have time to heal. Relax and let your energy go toward helping you heal.

· · · ·

# DEPRESSION

There are many mood disorders, depression being one. People who are chronically depressed should seek a diagnosis from a professional to ensure they are not suffering from clinical depression, which is extremely serious and does require medical intervention. There can be many reasons or no discernable reason at all for depression. Sometimes we have very valid reasons to be depressed, but it is those times when we can't exactly put our finger on our feelings of sadness that are worrisome to us. Depression hurts not only the person feeling depressed, but their loved ones, their career, their friendships, their health, and all facets of life. Essential oils, Ayurveda, herbs, and home remedies have been used for thousands of years as a way of dispelling the feelings of doom and gloom often associated with depression.

## AYURVEDA: *Depression Approach*

Ayurveda teaches us that when we are in a state of depression, everything is involved: our mind, spirit, body, doshas, and essentially everything we are made up of is out of balance. Some Ayurvedic tips to get back into balance following depression include:

- A healthy diet is on the menu when struggling with depression. Some of the foods that will counteract depression are plenty of fresh fruits, vegetables, fruit juices, and water. Do not eat processed foods when depressed as they will weigh the body down, clog up the thought processes, and lead to negative thinking.

- Combine equal amounts of the following spices in a jar and sprinkle on food such as salads, casseroles, and vegetables to lift the spirits and banish depression: cumin, turmeric, powdered ginger, minced and dried rosemary, and black pepper. Keep the jar in a cool, dark area for up to one year.

- Try to think positively. Only associate with positive people when possible. When negative thoughts intrude, gently swat them aside and replace them with happy memories or goals. The hardest task in the world is trying to control our thoughts, but with much-needed practice, it begins to be easier to banish the negative and instill the positive.

## HERB: *Euphoria Salve*

These herbs have a great reputation for dispelling gloom and restoring good mental health and are full of antidepressants and energy-promoting properties. I like to keep this salve around during hard and troubling times in my life. I use it daily to promote positive thoughts and push away negative thoughts.

½ CUP ST. JOHN'S WORT

½ CUP GINGKO BILOBA

½ CUP CHAMOMILE

1 CUP OLIVE OR SESAME OIL

1 OUNCE BEESWAX

½ TEASPOON VITAMIN E OIL

Pack the herbs into the olive or sesame oil and cook on very low heat on stovetop for 1½ hours, stirring occasionally. Strain through cheesecloth into a glass bowl, add beeswax, and stir until beeswax is melted. Add vitamin E and stir. Pour a drop of the mixture onto the counter. Run your finger through the drop after a few seconds of cooling: if it is too thick, add a little oil; if it is too thin, add a little more beeswax. Once you are happy with the consistency, pour into a jar and label. Cool before applying to areas such as wrists, neck, chest, or temples by rubbing or massaging into the skin. Store in a cool, dark area for up to one year.

## ESSENTIAL OIL: *Joyful Salt Bath*

These essential oils pack a powerful, happy punch. To help us lift that depressed feeling, this bath salt blend contains therapeutic properties including antidepressant, euphoric, nervine, and aphrodisiacal elements. These jars make attractive, inexpensive, and healing gifts!

9 DROPS LAVENDER OIL

7 DROPS NEROLI OIL

7 DROPS FRANKINCENSE OIL

4 DROPS YLANG-YLANG OIL

1 TABLESPOON CARRIER OIL (SUCH AS JOJOBA, SESAME, GRAPESEED, OR YOUR PREFERENCE)

3 CUPS SALT (PINK HIMALAYAN, SEA, EPSOM, OR YOUR PREFERENCE)

1 TABLESPOON MILK (OPTIONAL)

Add the essential oils and carrier oil to salt. Stir until essential oil and salt mixture are well blended. Cover tightly. Leave mixture in a dark area for twenty-four hours, then stir mixture again. Run the bathwater, but not so hot as to ruin the oils. Add a half cup of the bath salt mixture to bathwater. If you add milk to the water, it will prevent the oil from floating on top of the water and sticking to your skin. Store remainder in a glass jar with a tight-fitting lid in a cool, dark area for up to three months.

## HOME REMEDY: *Uplifting Rice Bake*

This healthy vegetarian rice dish is full of foods that lift the spirits and diminish those melancholy blues. Science has shown that saffron, asparagus, pumpkin seeds, citrus, and several other foods have nutrients to help combat depression.

1 CUP COOKED BASMATI RICE

¼ CUP CHOPPED MUSHROOMS

¼ CUP CHOPPED ONIONS

1 TABLESPOON BUTTER (OR GHEE)

½ CUP VEGETABLE BROTH

½ CUP MILK

1 BUNCH ASPARAGUS, WASHED AND CHOPPED

1 BOILED EGG, DICED

3–5 SAFFRON NEEDLES

½ TEASPOON LEMON JUICE

¼ TEASPOON SALT

1 TEASPOON ROASTED PUMPKIN SEEDS

Pour cooked rice into a greased casserole dish. Sauté the mushrooms and onion in the butter for three minutes, then add to cooked rice. Add all of the remaining ingredients to the rice and stir. Cover with foil. Bake for twenty minutes. Remove foil and cook until bubbly and thick, about ten to fifteen minutes. Serve with salad and a protein such as fish or added nuts. Store remainder in refrigerator for up to two days.

• • • •

# DETOX

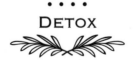

When you are ridding the body of substances that are harmful to your well-being or just giving yourself a good cleaning out, detox can be the ultimate path to take. Detox can be used to get the body refreshed and invigorated after a time of eating unhealthy food. Detox can also assist a person who wants to stop drinking alcohol, partaking in drugs, or smoking cigarettes. Just as there are various techniques used throughout the world to help people remain calm, centered, and focused throughout the process, there are numerous natural detoxifying elements to help with your detoxification regimen.

## AYURVEDA: *Detox Oil Pull*

This oil pull uses oils that have been utilized forever for their detoxifying elements. I like to use this when I am trying to get germs and chemicals out of my body; they are attracted to the oil and expelled. I end up with a clean and positive experience each time I complete this ritual.

½ TEASPOON SESAME OIL

½ TEASPOON SUNFLOWER OIL

Add the oils to a large spoon. Place the spoonful of oils into the mouth. Very gently, swish oil between all teeth, over tongue, and in all areas of the mouth for ten to fifteen minutes. After you are done, spit all of the oil out of your mouth and into the garbage. Do not swallow the oil. Repeat every morning for two weeks.

## HERB: *Nettle Detox Decoction*

This is the first decoction that I ever drank. I used it as a tonic for overall health and well-being. I liked it so much and felt so good that I have enjoyed it many times since.

¼ CUP DANDELION LEAVES

¼ CUP PEPPERMINT LEAVES

¼ CUP NETTLE

1 QUART WATER

Place the dried herbs in a quart-size mason jar. Boil water and fill up jar with the boiling water. Seal tightly and let steep for eight to ten hours (make at night and let set until morning). Strain and discard herbs. If desired, add honey or sweetener, stir, and drink throughout the day. Drink a cup or two daily for best effect. Store in refrigerator in a jar with a tight-fitting lid for up to twenty-four hours.

## ESSENTIAL OIL: *Detoxifying Massage Oil*

Using this massage oil will add detoxifying essential oils throughout the body. The massage you receive will calm your mind and bring peace as you go through the withdrawal process. Stay focused on the positive regarding how much better your life will be without the chemicals in your body.

12 DROPS HONEYSUCKLE OIL

10 DROPS ANGELICA OIL

8 DROPS PEPPERMINT OIL

6 DROPS VITAMIN E OIL

½ OUNCE CARRIER OIL (SESAME AND GRAPESEED ARE GREAT FOR THIS)

Mix ingredients in a glass container and lightly massage the area desired, such as temples, neck, chest, back, or soles of feet. Keep essential oil mixture away from open wounds, mucus membranes, genitals, eyes, and sensitive areas. Repeat application as needed. Store unused portion in a glass jar with a tight-fitting lid, label it, and keep it in a cool, dark area for up to three months.

## HOME REMEDY: *Detox Grocery List*

Many foods have natural detoxifying properties. Add these foods to your grocery shopping list the next time you wish to detoxify your body. These foods help to restore pH balance back to normal, calm the mind, ease stomach issues, and rid the body of toxins. Make a salad of several of the following ingredients and add a splash of apple cider vinegar as the dressing:

- apple, banana, beet, carrot, cayenne pepper, celery, dandelion, flaxseed, grapefruit, kale, lemon, lettuce, lime, orange, parsley, spinach, turmeric

. . . .

# DIARRHEA

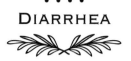

When the bowels are overactive, this can cause several uncomfortable and even painful symptoms such as bloating, nausea, cramping, and gas. People all over the world have used a host of remedies to put an end to this uncomfortable and sometimes dangerous condition. Diarrhea is not only aggravating, but it can often be indicative of more serious issues. If diarrhea is chronic, seek medical treatment. Diarrhea can lead to dehydration, so ensure that you are staying hydrated by drinking an excess of water. Try a few of these recipes and tips the next time you have diarrhea and see which one works best for you.

### AYURVEDA: *Rice Preparation*

This calming, soothing recipe will be gentle enough to ease diarrhea but medicinally powerful enough to restore balance throughout the digestive tract. Make up a batch of this next time you have diarrhea and eat small portions five to six times daily until digestion is under control.

½ CUP BASMATI RICE

1 CUP WATER

1 TABLESPOON GHEE

¼ TEASPOON GINGER

½ APPLE, DICED

YOGURT (OPTIONAL)

Prepare the rice according to package directions. During the last five minutes of cooking, add the ghee, ginger, and diced apples. You may add yogurt to the final dish if you desire.

### HERB: *Ginger Mint Tea*

This remedy just sounds like it will help because we know how good these herbs are for digestive issues. We all have used ginger and peppermint at various times in our lives to ease stomach upset and diarrhea. Sipping on this will calm the bowels and restore order downstairs.

1 CUP WATER

1 TABLESPOON GRATED GINGER

1 TABLESPOON PEPPERMINT LEAVES

Bring water to a boil, then add herbs. Remove from heat, cover, and steep for six to eight minutes. Strain and, if desired, add sweetener of choice. Compost or discard herbs.

## ESSENTIAL OIL: *The Stopper Oils*

This is the main recipe I use. It is soothing and helps my bowels and muscles calm down with its antispasmodic and pain-relieving properties.

8 DROPS GINGER OIL

8 DROPS PEPPERMINT OIL

8 DROPS CYPRESS OIL

½ OUNCE CARRIER OIL (SUCH AS JOJOBA, SESAME, GRAPESEED, OR YOUR PREFERENCE)

5 DROPS VITAMIN E OIL

Mix the ingredients in a small glass container and apply lightly to the area desired, such as lower back and abdomen. Keep essential oil mixture away from open wounds, mucus membranes, genitals, eyes, and sensitive areas. Repeat application as needed, usually two to three times daily. Store unused portion in a glass jar with a tight-fitting lid, label it, and keep it in a cool, dark area for up to six months.

## HOME REMEDY: *Diarrhea Tips*

These tips below have been used throughout the world during the last several thousand years for diarrhea. These are easy to incorporate into daily life for children as well as adults. Bring healing and comfort with a few of these tips.

- Drink plenty of water to help flush toxins from the body.

- Blackberries, bananas, and applesauce help heal the colon and rid the body of viruses that are causing the diarrhea.

- Yogurt restores balance and rids the body of bad bacteria in the stomach that is responsible for the diarrhea.

- Dairy products will ferment in the stomach and cause more issues in the bowels.

- Include rice, toast, and crackers in small amounts. Eat several small meals during the day rather than a couple of large meals. It is easier for the body to digest tiny portions.

· · · ·

# DIGESTIVE ISSUES

Diet, disease, illness, stress, spicy foods, allergies, heredity—the list of why a person suffers from digestive issues is endless. Taking care of yourself is the first order of business. Unwinding, eating healthy, and consulting medical specialists are priorities when dealing with chronic digestive issues. So many people think that digestive issues are a part of life and become accustomed to dealing with it. In Ayurveda it is believed that all illness stems from the digestive tract. Keeping your digestion in good running order is paramount to good total body health. Below are some of the recipes used worldwide to help get that digestive system running at peak performance.

### AYURVEDA: *Digestive Tips*

In Ayurvedic medicine, digestive issues always lead to a more serious condition elsewhere in the body. To keep the rest of the body in tip-top shape, you should always concentrate on healing any digestive issues first. Here are a few tips on how to keep stomach, colon, and bowels running efficiently and smoothly.

- Drink one teaspoon apple cider vinegar daily or add to a salad. Vinegar is a natural probiotic that will increase good bacteria and destroy bad bacteria.

- Eat a piece of licorice every day to keep your stomach feeling at its peak and to keep digestion flowing properly.

- Probiotics are a great supplement for good bacteria in the digestive tract.

- Eat several small meals a day instead of two or three large meals. This is easier on the digestive system and will help restore natural balance.

- Exercise assists in keeping the digestive system at its peak performance. It helps move things around so that your food doesn't sit in one area and ferment.

- Drink tepid water. Room-temperature drinks are ideal when dealing with stomach issues. Ice tends to slow down digestion, and heat causes fermentation.

- A positive attitude goes a long way in dealing with issues such as ulcers and stomach tension. Try to focus on peaceful, happy thoughts.

- Do not eat after 7 or 8 pm. Try to set a schedule for meals that you can follow and not deviate from.

- Eat a piece of ginger with salt on it when stomach issues first start. Ginger is very calming for the digestive tract.

- Meditate and pray daily to bring peace to your soul and end stress in your life. Stress has been shown to play a major role in digestive issues, and science has proven that meditation is an optimal pain reliever.

## HERB: *Digestive Infusion*

Infusions are like strong teas, ideal for herbal blends that contain seeds or woody stems. This infusion is great to sip throughout the day to relieve a plethora of stomach and digestive issues. The anti-inflammatory and anti-spasmodic properties settle the digestive tract and help to reduce nausea, acid reflux, bloating, cramping, and other digestive issues.

1 TEASPOON FENNEL SEEDS

1 TABLESPOON GRATED GINGER

2 TABLESPOONS LEMON BALM LEAVES

1 TABLESPOON CHAMOMILE FLOWERS

2 CUPS BOILING WATER

Place herbs in a mason jar. Pour the hot water over the herbs and leave eight to ten hours or overnight. Strain and, if desired, add sweetener of choice. Compost or discard herbs. Drink one to two cups daily. Refrigerate any remainder for up to forty-eight hours.

## ESSENTIAL OIL: *Tummy Rub*

Stomachic properties abound in these essential oils. This tummy rub has anti-spasmodic and anti-inflammatory properties to heal your digestive tract and minimize symptoms.

> 10 DROPS CHAMOMILE OIL
>
> 10 DROPS FENNEL OIL
>
> 6 DROPS ANISE OIL
>
> 5 DROPS VITAMIN E OIL
>
> ½ OUNCE CARRIER OIL (SUCH AS JOJOBA, SESAME, GRAPESEED, OR YOUR PREFERENCE)

Mix the ingredients in a small glass container and apply lightly to the area desired, such as abdomen and lower back. Keep essential oil mixture away from open wounds, mucus membranes, genitals, eyes, and sensitive areas. Repeat application as needed, usually two to three times daily. Store unused portion in a glass jar with a tight-fitting lid, label it, and keep it in a cool, dark area for up to six months.

## HOME REMEDY: *Digestive Juice*

This drink is full of anti-inflammatory and anti-spasmodic properties. Drink daily until your body is feeling better and your symptoms are gone. The healing properties in these foods help to clean out your digestive tract, restore order to your stomach and colon, and give you a great overall feeling.

> 1 STALK CELERY
>
> 1 HANDFUL KALE LEAVES
>
> 1 TEASPOON FENNEL SEEDS
>
> 1 APPLE, CORED
>
> ½-INCH GINGER ROOT

Combine all of the ingredients into a juicer or blender. Add enough water or herbal tea to get the mixture to the consistency you like to drink. Drink throughout the day each day for two weeks. You should notice a big improvement in your digestion issues. Store remainder in the refrigerator for up to twenty-four hours.

· · · ·

# EARACHE

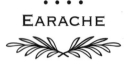

There is nothing worse than that throbbing ear pain. This can be caused by water in the ear, wax buildup, blowing the nose often, or a variety of reasons. If fever is present, seek medical attention for a diagnosis to ensure infection is not present.

### AYURVEDA: *Earache Drop*

These two ingredients together are miracle workers in the world of Ayurveda. Try a drop or two of this blend and you will find yourself quickly on the way to health.

1 PULVERIZED GARLIC CLOVE

1 TABLESPOON SESAME OIL

Add the finely mashed garlic clove to the sesame oil and cook on low heat on the stovetop for two to three minutes. Let cool for a few minutes until very mildly warm. Strain the oil and discard the garlic. Place one or two drops in an eye dropper and drip into ear. Hold head at angle so it will not run out for about four minutes. Repeat on other side as needed. Remove any of the oil that runs out of the ear with a swab. Remainder may be kept at room temperature in a container with a tight-fitting lid for up to twenty-four hours. Repeat process every six hours.

## HERB: *Elderberry Syrup*

Elderberries not only taste so good but are full of pain-relieving and healing properties. Try a spoonful of this syrup three to five times daily to reduce pain and speed up the healing process of an earache.

**3 CUPS WATER**

**½ CUP ELDERBERRIES, DRIED**

**4 TABLESPOONS LEMON JUICE**

**3 TABLESPOONS HONEY**

Pour water in a pan and bring to a boil. Add the elderberries and reduce heat to low. Cover and heat until almost half of the water is gone. Remove from heat; leave covered and steep for one hour. Strain liquid, discard berries, add lemon juice and honey while liquid is still hot; stir. Add more honey until it reaches desired thickness. Cool and place in bottle. Adults get one tablespoon and children one teaspoon as needed. Store in refrigerator for up to one week.

## ESSENTIAL OIL: *Ear Swab*

These oils have antispasmodic, analgesic, and anti-inflammatory properties to help heal and soothe an earache.

**2 DROPS GINGER OIL**

**2 DROPS PEPPERMINT OIL**

**1 COTTON SWAB**

Combine the oils into a small bowl. Dip one end of the cotton swab into the mixture. Swipe the outer ear canal with the oils. Do not get directly into the ear canal. Essential oils are concentrated and can burn or cause damage if placed into the ear without dilution. Use mixture for up to twenty-four hours to receive healing and pain-reducing benefits. You can place a drop or two on a cotton ball and insert slightly inside ear for instant relief.

I remember going to school often as a child with a cotton ball stuck in my ear. Just the air movement around my ear would cause pain, so the cotton ball was a good old friend and the oil helped to loosen hardened wax. Try this to bring some comfort to someone with an earache—they will thank you.

**3 DROPS OLIVE OIL**

**1 COTTON BALL**

Pour the olive oil onto one side of the cotton ball. Place the wet side first into the ear opening. Do not push or shove into the ear canal. The olive oil helps to soften any hardened ear wax, making it easy to remove with a swab. Leave in place for eight hours or overnight, then replace if desired with a new cotton ball and oil.

· · · ·

# ECZEMA (DERMATITIS AND SKIN ISSUES)

Eczema and dermatitis outbreaks run rampant in my family. We have traced it to wheat, dairy, nightshades, and sugar. (Sounds like a recipe for a cake, right?) Discovering what causes skin flare-ups is a tedious job. It is usually food or chemical related. Stress can cause a flare-up to happen, but food and chemicals are the main culprits and cause the allergy to just wait beneath the skin for a reason to come out! The elimination diet is the perfect way to abstain from certain foods and find out what is the root of the problem. Below are a few of the ways that people around the world bring relief to these uncomfortable, painful, unsightly ailments.

**AYURVEDA: *Turmeric Paste***

Turmeric has many cicatrisant and vulnerary properties to heal all types of skin ailments. Use this paste often throughout several days and you will put an end to that outbreak fast.

**1 TABLESPOON TURMERIC**

**1 TABLESPOON SESAME OIL**

Combine the two ingredients together well. Apply paste to desired area and cover with a bandage or gauze. Turmeric will stain clothing and furniture if not covered. Leave on for several hours. Wash site well and reapply as needed. Remainder may be covered and refrigerated for up to three days.

## HERB: *Soothing Skin Poultice*

The cicatrisant properties of chamomile have a gentle healing effect on skin outbreaks. Use this wash as often as desired to bring about relief and comfort to those painful outbreaks.

½ CUP CHAMOMILE FLOWERS

2 CUPS BOILING WATER

LINEN OR CLOTH

Place the herbs into the boiling water. Remove from heat, cover, and steep for about half an hour. Strain and discard herbs. Drench a piece of linen or cloth into the mixture and either place cloth on skin and leave until temperature is uncomfortable or wash onto skin and allow to air-dry. Repeat process throughout the day. Discard mixture after twenty-four hours.

## ESSENTIAL OIL: *Fresh Eczema Rub*

This rub has anti-inflammatory, emollient, and cicatrisant properties to moisturize and heal many outbreaks. Apply several times daily to promote healing and prevent further cracks and sores.

10 DROPS CALENDULA OIL

10 DROPS FRANKINCENSE OIL

10 DROPS TEA TREE OIL

5 DROPS PALMAROSA OIL

1 OUNCE CARRIER OIL (SUCH AS JOJOBA, SESAME, GRAPESEED, OR YOUR PREFERENCE)

5 DROPS VITAMIN E OIL

Mix the ingredients in a small glass container and apply lightly to the desired area. Keep essential oil mixture away from open wounds, mucus membranes, genitals, eyes, and sensitive areas. Repeat application as needed, Store unused portion in a glass jar with a tight-fitting lid, label it, and keep it in a cool, dark area for up to six months.

**HOME REMEDY:** *Oatmeal Bath Skin Sachet*

This is an age-old remedy for any type of skin issue. Oatmeal has healing properties and soothing components that help to heal and soothe itchy, dry skin. I like to use this sachet to give my skin an overall glow and add a spa feel to my bath.

1 CHEESECLOTH SQUARE

½ CUP OATS (NOT INSTANT)

½ FOOT STRING OR RIBBON

Lay the cheesecloth flat. Place the oats in the middle of the cloth, bring up all of the edges together, and tie a ribbon around the middle of the gathered edges so that all of the oatmeal is in a little ball in the middle of the material. Place the sachet in the bath water and let the properties of the oatmeal dissipate into the water. You can grasp the ball by the gathered edge and rub the oatmeal over your entire body or just over the breakout area. When you are done, discard the sachet. This keeps the oats from clogging up your drain, but you still receive all of the benefits of an oatmeal bath!

• • • •

# ENERGY

We all need it, we all want it, but energy can sometimes be so fleeting. Having enough energy to get through our hectic, busy lives is paramount to our good living. Taking care of one's self from the inside out is vital to keeping our energy up day after day. Sometimes we just don't have the energy we need, so we look to other sources. Before you turn to chemicals and caffeine, try a few of these natural alternative recipes from around the world to naturally get your energy back up to par.

## AYURVEDA: *Super Drink*

This Ayurvedic drink will give you vitamins, minerals, and therapeutic properties to keep your energy at an all-time high. This morning wake-me-up is consumed by people all over the world daily. Enjoy this drink at room temperature, the Ayurvedic way!

½ TEASPOON GHEE

1 CUP MILK

4 ALMONDS, CRUSHED

1 DATE, CHOPPED

1 PIECE GINSENG, GRATED

1 SAFFRON NEEDLE

HONEY (OPTIONAL)

Bring ghee, milk, almonds, date, and ginseng to a low boil. Remove from heat and add the saffron. Stir, cover, and let sit until desired temperature. Strain and discard pieces into compost heap, reserving the milk. Add honey to taste to the milk (optional). Drink in the morning for an increased level of energy throughout the day. Refrigerate remainder for up to twenty-four hours.

## HERB: *Energy Tea*

Wow! Talk about packing a punch. This tea will give you the needed energy to accomplish everything on your to-do list. Make enough to last all day and drink it hot or over ice. Hot or cold, this tea will be just the boost you need.

1 CUP WATER

½-INCH PIECE GINSENG, CHOPPED

1 TABLESPOON NETTLE

1 TEASPOON HOLY BASIL LEAVES

1 TEASPOON YERBA MATE

Bring water to a boil, then add herbs. Remove from heat, cover, and steep for ten to twelve minutes. Strain and, if desired, add sweetener of choice. Compost or discard herbs.

## ESSENTIAL OIL: *Energy Diffuser*

This is the recipe I run most often on days I want to stay home and clean, cook, write, and take care of my responsibilities and tasks. Just smelling these aromas in the air can give me the boost I need to get up and go!

**5 DROPS PEPPERMINT OIL**

**4 DROPS LEMONGRASS OIL**

**3 DROPS PINE OIL**

**WATER**

Add oils and water to diffuser and run as desired.

## HOME REMEDY: *Energetic Tips*

Here are a few common-sense hints and tips to keep energy levels up for the long run. Practicing these tips each day will get you healthier and more energetic overall.

- Take multivitamins daily or at least vitamin B. Drink milk, which has vitamin B and D in it as well.

- Juice each day with a multitude of fruits and vegetables, especially spinach and kale. All kinds of healing and energy-inducing effects come with juicing.

- It may be hard to believe that working out can give you energy, but it is a proven fact. Have you ever been exhausted from just sitting around all day? Movement creates energy. Take a walk. Practice yoga. Swim. Any type of exercise will be beneficial for you.

- Stress can not only make you ill, it can zap your energy. Meditate, pray, listen or play music, read, write. Anything you find that can help you to remove negative energy and replace it with positive energy will benefit you overall.

- Hydrate! Water is the most life-giving force on earth. The more you drink, the better off you will be mentally and physically.

- Eat low calorie, lowfat meals. Eat small meals so that all of your energy won't go toward digesting large meals. Lots of fruits and vegetables are the number-one source of energy for our bodies.

• • • •
# Eyestrain

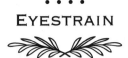

Computers, cell phones, and continuous straining of the eye muscles often leave you with a tired, achy feeling in your eyes. If you suffer from eyestrain chronically, then you should visit an ophthalmologist to ensure no other issues exist.

### AYURVEDA: *Yoga Eyestrain Asanas*

In Ayurveda it is believed that the best way to get over eyestrain is to exercise the eye muscles. Try these poses daily to get stronger eyes.

Sit in a comfortable chair or on the floor with your legs crossed. Place hands, palms up and relaxed, on the knees. Sit with back straight and head in a comfortable, straight position. Rotate eyes, without moving head, to stare up at ceiling or sky. Hold position for two breaths. Rotate eyes, without moving head, to stare far right, and hold for two breaths. Rotate eyes, without moving head, to stare far left, and hold for two breaths. Rotate eyes, without moving head, to stare down toward chin, and hold for two breaths. Bring eyes straight forward, without moving head, and close eyes. Hold for two breaths. Two times a day, repeat entire process twice.

### HERB: *Eye Poultice*

Green tea has antioxidants that fight all sorts of eye disorders as well as eyestrain. This age-old poultice feels so soothing and will have your eyes feeling great in just a couple of minutes.

**2 GREEN TEA BAGS**

**1 CUP BOILING WATER**

**LINEN OR CLOTH**

Place the herbs into 1 cup of boiling water. Remove from heat, cover, and steep for six to eight minutes, then strain and cool (can be refrigerated for quicker cooling). Using a piece of linen or cloth, soak material in the tea. Apply the cloth to closed eyes and relax. Do not apply to mucus membranes, open eyeballs, genitals, open wounds, or other sensitive areas. Change as cloth temperature becomes uncomfortable. Reapply as often as needed. Discard any remaining tea.

## ESSENTIAL OIL: *Oil Massage Eye Rub*

Several essential oils have therapeutic properties that soothe, heal, and comfort the eyes. Using this rub on the outer eyelids and eye sockets will bring rapid relief, but do not get these oils directly on your eyeball.

2 DROPS HELICHRYSUM

2 DROPS FRANKINCENSE

½ TEASPOON CARRIER OIL (SUCH AS JOJOBA, SESAME, GRAPESEED, OR YOUR PREFERENCE)

2 DROPS VITAMIN E OIL

In a small bowl or container, mix the ingredients together with a small whisk. Using fingertips, rub onto closed eyelids and around eye sockets, upper cheeks, and forehead areas. Do not apply mixture to mucus membranes, open eyes, genitals, mouth, wounds, or sensitive areas. Rub area desired with a circular motion until the skin absorbs the mixture. When done with massage, wipe off excess with a towel.

## HOME REMEDY: *Old-Time Eye Soother*

This is an easy, quick, effective way to bring comfort and relief to aching, tired eyes.

1 TEASPOON WITCH HAZEL

2 COTTON BALLS

Pour half of the witch hazel onto each of the cotton balls. Be sure to do this over an area that is easy to clean up in the event any liquid spills. Place the soaked cotton balls over the closed eyelids and allow to rest on eyelids. Lie back and keep this quiet position for about five minutes. Do not get any of the mixture onto the eyeballs. After you are done, wipe excess moisture from eyes. Ahhhh … now *that's* a good feeling!

· · · ·
# FEVER

The body has many abilities, and most of them we are not even aware of. One of these abilities is to turn up the heat to burn out viruses and kill foreign invaders such as infections. The body's furnace-burning, infection-killing heat is also known as fever. Not only can our fevers burn up and kill foreign invaders in our body, if prolonged or too high, fever can kill us as well. Fever can range from slight and uncomfortable to debilitating or deadly. If fever is present for a long period or too high, seek medical attention immediately.

## AYURVEDA: *Fever Sipper*

It has been said that you can smell this drink all over India during the flu and cold seasons. These ingredients contain everything you need to fight a mild fever and, in most cases, eliminate it altogether. The taste may not be to your liking, but the results will be!

½ CUP WATER

2 GARLIC CLOVES, MINCED

½ TEASPOON TURMERIC

½ TEASPOON HONEY

1 SLICE LEMON

Heat water to boiling on the stove. Add the garlic and turn down heat to low. Cook for five minutes. Strain and discard garlic pieces. Add the turmeric, honey, and lemon. Cool to room temperature. Drink slowly, one spoonful at a time, over the course of the day. Discard any remainder.

## HERB: *Fever Tincture*

This tincture has febrifuge, sedative, and healing properties to bring down a fever quickly and rid the body of the germs that caused the fever. Drink two to three spoonfuls two to three times daily for optimal results. This recipe takes six weeks to make, so make it ahead of time, and it will last through several seasons.

3 TABLESPOONS YARROW LEAVES

2 TABLESPOONS CHAMOMILE FLOWERS

2 TABLESPOONS PEPPERMINT LEAVES

2 TABLESPOONS LEMON BALM

¾ PINT VEGETABLE GLYCERIN OR VODKA

Place herbs in a pint jar until it's half full with dried herbs or two-thirds full with fresh herbs, and cover the herbs with a high proof vodka (for adults) or vegetable glycerin (for children), about an inch from the top of the jar. Cover tightly and place in a cool, dark location. Shake vigorously every day for two weeks, and then let it set without shaking for one month. Strain, bottle, label and put the date you decanted it (strained the herb). Use ½–1 dropperful in tea, water, or other liquid. Store in a cool, dark area in a jar with a tight-fitting lid for up to three years (vodka) or one year (glycerin).

## ESSENTIAL OIL: *Cool Oil Spray*

This spray is loaded with cooling elements, healing agents, and febrifuge properties. Use this on face or body as often as you wish to help reduce fever and cool the body.

10 DROPS EUCALYPTUS OIL

10 DROPS PEPPERMINT OIL

10 DROPS NIAOULI OIL

2 OUNCES WATER

1 TEASPOON WITCH HAZEL

Add all ingredients to a dark-colored spray bottle to prevent sunlight from damaging contents. Shake bottle and spray onto area desired, such as body, face, legs, or chest. Do not spray into open wounds, genitals, eyes, or mucus membranes. Store in a cool, dark area for up to three months. Shake well before each use to combine the ingredients.

## HOME REMEDY: *Fever Remedies*

These home remedies are easy to do and effective. When trying to rid someone of a low fever, try incorporating a few of these practices throughout the day to help them reduce that fever and feel better. If fever is very high or persistent, it is better to seek professional medical treatment.

- Take a lukewarm bath. The cooler water will help to bring down the body temperature. (For adults only!)

- Ice packs or cool cloths to the forehead for twenty minutes. It might be uncomfortable, but this practice has worked for generations.

- Drink as much water or vitamin-enhanced drinks as possible throughout the day. Fever tends to dehydrate the body very rapidly.

- Take vitamin C or drink juices that are rich in vitamin C.

- No meat, chocolate, or dairy. These foods will unsettle the stomach. Eat light crackers, broth, gelatin, or mild soups.

- Drink herbal teas. There are many herbs that have febrifuge properties, and the liquid will help with the hydration process.

- A good treat for children, while reducing fever at the same time, is frozen popsicles. They taste great, and kids don't have to know it's for medicinal purposes!

· · · ·

# FLU

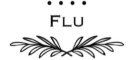

The flu causes such a wide range of symptoms—from aches, pains, sore throat, chills, fever, stomach issues, headache, coughing, and it goes on and on. Below are a few of the remedies practiced around the world to get you back on your feet and in tip-top shape again.

AYURVEDA: *Digestive Flu Broth*

This Ayurvedic recipe is great for the stomach flu. It has stomachic and nausea-fighting properties to help heal and calm the digestive tract. It also has a pleasing taste and is easy on the stomach for someone who can't eat due to nausea.

**1 CUP BROTH**

**½-INCH GINGER ROOT, MINCED**

**2 GARLIC CLOVES, MINCED**

**1 TEASPOON TURMERIC**

Heat the broth to boiling on the stove. Lower heat to simmer and add the ginger and the garlic. Heat for five to ten minutes. Remove from heat and cool slightly, until warm enough to eat. Add the turmeric, stir, and enjoy. Any remainder may be refrigerated for up to twenty-four hours.

**HERB:** *Flu Super Herbal Syrup*

This syrup has every healing property for symptoms associated with the flu. It tastes great and is really fun to make. When my kids were young, this was about the only herbal remedy I made that they didn't complain about when they had to take it. Set aside one hour before the flu season to make this up. It will last quite a while.

**¾ CUP ELDERBERRIES**

**4 CUPS FILTERED WATER**

**1 CUP HONEY**

Put the elderberries in a pan and cover with the water. Bring to a boil, then lower heat and simmer for an hour or until the liquid is reduced by half. Remove from heat and cool slightly. Mash the elderberries into the water mixture. Pour through a strainer and discard berries. When the mixture has cooled, add the honey and whisk well. This syrup may be placed in a jar with a tight-fitting lid, labeled, and refrigerated for up to one month.

**ESSENTIAL OIL:** *Flu Roll-On*

This roll-on is the perfect flu fighter. It is easy to carry, easy to use, and full of the therapeutic properties you need to fight the flu. Some of these components include antibacterial, antibiotic, anti-infective, anti-inflammatory, decongestant, expectorant, and sudorific agents.

**8 DROPS EUCALYPTUS OIL**

**8 DROPS THYME OIL**

**6 DROPS PEPPERMINT OIL**

**5 DROPS OREGANO OIL**

**½ OUNCE CARRIER OIL (SUCH AS JOJOBA, SESAME, GRAPESEED, OR YOUR PREFERENCE)**

**4 DROPS VITAMIN E OIL**

Combine the ingredients into a small bowl. Pour into one or two roll-on bottles. Adjust cap accordingly and label the bottles. Roll onto desired areas such as temples, neck, back, chest, or soles of feet. This particular recipe is good for both digestive or respiratory flu. Keep in cool, dark area for up to six months.

**HOME REMEDY:** *Old Mustard Foot Bath*

Many home remedies are directed toward the feet to heal the flu. It is believed that heating up the feet will get the blood pumping throughout the entire body and will direct the blood to specific areas to heal, break up congestion, and get the foggy brain working again. This recipe targets the feet, not only heating them with water but with mustard, which has very hot properties as well as circulatory agents to work in getting that blood going.

**1½ TABLESPOONS DRY MUSTARD POWDER**

**1½ QUARTS HOT WATER**

Mix the two ingredients into a pan or bowl that will accommodate your feet. When the water is at a temperature that will not burn or scald your feet, place your feet into the water mixture and sit back and relax. Keep your feet in the foot bath for about fifteen minutes or until the water cools. Repeat process one or two times daily until flu is gone. Discard water after each use.

• • • •

# FUNGUS

Several illnesses, incidents, and needs can bring an attack of fungal bacteria to a person or place. This red, scaly, itchy section of skin can be caused by a host of factors. Getting rid of it usually takes weeks, months, or even years. Try a few of these remedies from around the world to bring your fungal attacks under control.

### AYURVEDA: *Fungus Treatment*

In the East it is believed that to treat a fungus, you must treat the entire body and soul. Here are a few Ayurvedic treatments that are great advice for anyone with fungal issues. Many of these tips are just common-sense things we need to incorporate into our daily lives for overall great health.

- Eat plenty of leafy green vegetables and fruit such as melons, pears, plums, and apples. Stay away from all processed foods, sugar, wheat, dairy, meat, and frozen foods. Incorporate turmeric, garlic, ginseng, honey, lemon, and apple cider vinegar into your meals every day.

- Broths and herbal teas are especially good if you are suffering from any type of skin disorder. They not only hydrate your skin but often can have healing components that work like magic to kill fungus.

- We need lots of sunshine, vitamin D, and fresh air. Take a walk outside! If you don't feel like walking, getting out and sitting in a chair for ten minutes under the healing rays of the sun can do you and your skin a world of good.

- Yoga's sun salutation, stretching, forward bends, and lotus poses can all get your body and blood moving and take fresh blood to all areas of your skin. Take just five minutes to do a few of these asanas to help you have the blood pumping you need to fight a fungal infection.

### HERB: *Coconut Basil Fungus Paste*

Holy basil has many soothing and healing antifungal qualities. Mixed with coconut oil, you have a blend that will work overtime to get your skin back to its soft, healthy appearance.

**1 TEASPOON HOLY BASIL LEAVES**

**1 TABLESPOON COCONUT OIL**

Mash the basil with a pestle and mortar until it is a fine powder. Mix the coconut oil and the basil powder together until a green paste forms. Apply the paste to the fungal site and cover with a bandage or gauze. Leave on all day or night. Reapply every day until fungus is gone. Store any remainder in a tiny jar with a lid, labeled, for up to one week.

## ESSENTIAL OIL: *Fungus Oil Rub*

These fungi-fighting essential oils are soothing and healing. Using this blend will speed up the healing process and get your skin glowing again.

> 15 DROPS TEA TREE OIL
>
> 10 DROPS MYRRH OIL
>
> 5 DROPS NEEM OIL
>
> 1 OUNCE CARRIER OIL (SUCH AS JOJOBA, SESAME, GRAPESEED, OR YOUR PREFERENCE)
>
> 5 DROPS VITAMIN E OIL

Mix the ingredients in a small glass container and apply lightly to the area attacked by fungus. Keep essential oil mixture away from open wounds, mucus membranes, genitals, eyes, and sensitive areas. Repeat application as needed, usually two to three times daily. Store unused portion in a glass jar with a tight-fitting lid, label it, and keep it in a cool, dark area for up to six months.

## HOME REMEDY: *Yogurt Fungus Fighter*

Yogurt has been used for years to fight fungal infections with its skin-healing properties. Your digestion, skin, and blood will benefit greatly.

> 1 SMALL CONTAINER OF YOGURT
>
> 1 PLUM, DICED

Combine these ingredients together, eat, and enjoy!

• • • •

# HAIR LOSS

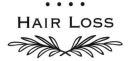

Losing your hair as you age is a natural progression of life. Losing too much hair at a young age can be devastating. The market is saturated with chemical products that claim to restore hair loss. Here I have listed several natural, non-chemical ways that people have strengthened their hair for thousands of years. You may want to give one of these a try before resorting to chemicals or surgery.

## AYURVEDA: *Hair Treatments*

In Ayurveda natural treatments always trump chemicals. Many of these treatments are practiced weekly or daily in India as a way to keep hair strong, shiny, and beautiful.

- Hair needs water to grow and remain healthy, so drink water every day.

- Inverted asanas (yoga poses with your head hanging down toward the floor) are good for getting blood to rush to your scalp and give new life to tired hair.

- It is believed in Ayurveda that too much pitta can lead to hair loss. In order to balance the pitta, one must follow a pitta diet, eat sweet fruits, and avoid hot, spicy, and salty foods. Eat asparagus. No alcohol or caffeine. Wear blue and purple to reduce pitta, and take cool showers.

- Make a hair wash out of a couple of hibiscus blooms and one teaspoon flaxseed in a half cup water. Let soak ten minutes. Strain, pour over scalp, and let sit for twenty minutes. Wash as usual.

- Make a tea of one teaspoon Indian gooseberry powder and one cup water. Pour on scalp and let sit fifteen minutes, then shampoo as usual.

## HERB: *Head Massage*

Rosemary has long been reported to restore hair loss and strengthen hair. First you need to make rosemary herbal oil, which is relatively easy to do. Once you have the oil, use it once weekly before you shampoo your hair.

¾ CUPS ROSEMARY NEEDLES, CHOPPED

1½ CUPS CARRIER OIL (SUCH AS JOJOBA, SESAME, GRAPESEED, OR YOUR PREFERENCE)

10 DROPS VITAMIN E OIL

Place rosemary in a jar and add the oils. Put the lid on the jar tightly, shake vigorously, and place jar in a cool, dark place. Shake every day for two weeks. Strain through cheesecloth, bottle, and label. Use two tablespoons oil as a scalp massage. Rub in for five to ten minutes, then wash hair as usual. Store for up to six months.

## ESSENTIAL OIL: *Strong Hair Shampoo*

Sage and chamomile have been known forever as oils that can have significant impact on the strength, luster, and growth of hair. Try adding these to your shampoo and see if you can bring new life back to your hair.

12-OUNCE BOTTLE OF SHAMPOO

10 DROPS VITAMIN E OIL

20 DROPS SAGE OIL (FOR BRUNETTES)

or

20 DROPS CHAMOMILE OIL (FOR BLONDES)

Mix the ingredients together in the shampoo bottle. Shake well before each use. Use as you normally would each time you shampoo your hair. Store shampoo bottle as you usually do, and it will last up to one year.

## HOME REMEDY: *Egg Wash*

This is a long-known remedy in North America, and it can work wonders on certain types of hair loss. At the least, it will shine and strengthen your hair.

1 EGG WHITE

2 TABLESPOONS OLIVE OIL

With a whisk, combine egg white and olive oil. Apply mixture by rubbing into the scalp until all areas are covered. Leave on for about twenty minutes, then wash hair as usual. Practice this method once weekly.

• • • •

# HANGOVER

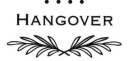

Hangovers are that head-pounding, nauseous, fatigued feeling you wake up with after a night of having too much fun. Alcohol affects all parts of the body, and boy do we pay for it. There are remedies-a-million for hangovers. Here are a few of the more practical ones.

### AYURVEDA: *Hangover Releaser*

This remedy is a favorite in India and all over the world. Get those nauseous, gassy feelings under control quickly with this powerful remedy and get your body back to normal.

> JUICE OF 1 LEMON
>
> 1 TABLESPOON BAKING SODA
>
> 1 CUP WATER

Mix all ingredients together into a cup and drink quickly. Discard any remainder.

### HERB: *Ginger Nausea Control*

Ginger is the ultimate tummy soother. Make this tea and sip it very slowly to dispel any queasy feelings.

> 1 CUP WATER
>
> ½-INCH GINGER ROOT, GRATED

Bring water to a boil, then add ginger. Remove from heat, cover, and steep for six to eight minutes. Strain and, if desired, add sweetener of choice. Compost or discard herbs.

### ESSENTIAL OIL: *Hangover Diffuser*

Getting these soothing, healing oils into the air may be your best bet to reducing those awful feelings associated with a hangover, both physical and mental. These oils have long been known to help with the morning after.

5 DROPS JUNIPER OIL

5 DROPS SANDALWOOD OIL

5 DROPS GRAPEFRUIT OIL

WATER

Add oils and water to diffuser and run as desired.

**HOME REMEDY:** *Hangover Juice Remedy*

All of the ingredients in this juice work well together to give you energy, dispel nausea, relieve a headache, and bring you back to normalcy.

1 CUP ORANGE JUICE

1 APPLE, CORED

1 BANANA

½ CUP ICE

1 PINCH SALT

½-INCH GINGER ROOT

Combine all ingredients into a blender or juicer. Blend. Drink throughout the day. Keep remainder in refrigerator for up to twenty-four hours.

• • • •

# HEADACHE

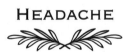

There are as many reasons for having a headache as there are stars in the sky. If pain is chronic or persistent, seek medical attention. Stress, overwork, worry, anxiety, illness, allergies, foods, heredity, and a host of reasons can cause a headache. People from every culture on earth have developed remedies to help end that excruciating pain so you can enjoy the world again.

**AYURVEDA:** *Headache Remedies*

Learning about which dosha you have as a primary is a very good exercise for anyone. Read the description of doshas on page 6 to spot which one is your primary. There are different headache remedies for each dosha. The following remedies are for all three dosha types: vata, pitta, and kapha.

- Squeeze the pad of flesh between the first and second toes for three to five minutes. This is a well-known acupressure technique practiced worldwide to relieve the pain of headaches.

- Try daily to incorporate some form of stress-relieving technique into your life. It has been shown that reducing stress could fully reduce 50 percent of the headaches in the world today.

- Drink water.

- Ensure that you get enough sleep each night. Make some bedtime rituals such as running a lavender diffuser or playing soft music that will get you in a restful frame of mind.

- Incorporating meditation and prayer into your life will reduce your stress so much. Meditation teaches us that we can overcome all types of pain. Prayer connects us to a higher power that we can rely on in times of pain.

- Once you discover which primary dosha you are, practice eating the diet that is best for balancing your primary dosha, as your diet can strongly affect your health. There are tons of good books and websites solely focused on what each dosha type needs.

- Chewing a piece of ginger root or drinking ginger tea significantly reduces headaches.

### HERB: *Headache Bath Sachet*

Lavender and peppermint have long been known to reduce headaches or eliminate them completely due to the anesthetic and vasodilator properties inherent in these herbs. This bath is relaxing, healing, and smells heavenly.

**¼ CUP LAVENDER FLOWERS**

**¼ CUP PEPPERMINT LEAVES**

**1 LINEN OR CHEESECLOTH SQUARE**

**1 FOOT RIBBON OR STRING**

Place the herbs in the center of the material and draw the edges up, forming a pocket. Using a string or ribbon, tie the edges of the material together, forming a ball of herbs at one end. Let this float in the bathtub as the water is running. The herbal oils will adhere to your cells and the aromas will permeate your senses, reducing headache. Discard herbs when bathing is completed.

## ESSENTIAL OIL: *Headache Rub*

Applying these oils to your head will have a calming, soothing action as the analgesic, anesthetic, antispasmodic, and anti-inflammatory properties work to alleviate your pain.

> **5 DROPS PATCHOULI OIL**
>
> **5 DROPS CAJEPUT OIL**
>
> **5 DROPS BERGAMOT OIL**
>
> **5 DROPS VITAMIN E OIL**
>
> **1 OUNCE CARRIER OIL (SUCH AS JOJOBA, SESAME, GRAPESEED, OR YOUR PREFERENCE)**

Mix the ingredients in a small glass container and apply lightly to the area desired, such as pressure points, neck, soles of feet, temples, and chest. Keep essential oil mixture away from open wounds, mucus membranes, genitals, eyes, and sensitive areas. Repeat application as needed, usually two to three times daily. Store unused portion in a glass jar with a tight-fitting lid, label it, and keep it in a cool, dark area for up to six months.

## HOME REMEDY: *Grannie's Headache Remedy*

If you tell your grannie that you have a headache, she is liable to spring into action using one of these time-tested techniques. Grannie knows what she is talking about, as the effects of these rituals have been scientifically proven to open blood vessels and allow that throbbing, dull pain to dissolve.

- Try crunching on almonds, as they are rife with components that enable your blood vessels to open and allow blood to pass through your throbbing temples quickly.

- Put a cold square of linen or a washcloth on your head as you lie still. Once this is no longer cold, take it off and replace it with a hot piece of linen. The action of hot followed by cold forces the blood vessels to constrict, then open alternately.

- Drink as much water as you can. Water thins the blood and allows it to flow more freely.

- Rub coconut oil onto your feet before bed. This will draw the blood away from your head and toward your feet.

• • • •

# HEARING LOSS

Hearing loss usually happens for a wide segment of the older population or is due to illness, heredity, disease, accidents, or many other reasons. Hearing loss can sometimes be reduced or even reversed with some of these recipes from around the world. Seeing a specialist to get a diagnosis on the problem with hearing can oftentimes lead to simple corrections, either through surgery, aids, or medications. If hearing loss is significant, it is imperative to get a professional opinion on how to proceed.

### AYURVEDA: *Hearing Diet*

In Ayurveda it is believed that hearing loss is caused primarily from poor liver function. Getting the liver back into good shape is the way to open the ears and increase hearing abilities. Diet plays a huge part in having optimal liver function. These Ayurvedic diet tips are to improve liver function and put an end to hearing loss.

- Eat small meals several times daily.
- Drink plenty of water.
- Reduce mucus by eliminating all dairy.
- Eat fish, chicken, beans, walnuts, eggs, and yams.
- Do not eat cold foods, cold drinks, or salads.

### HERB: *Ear Decoction*

This herbal remedy is hundreds of years old. Drinking these herbs has been reported to reduce stress, thereby increasing blood flow to the head and the ears in particular.

½ TEASPOON LEMON BALM LEAVES

¼ TEASPOON ROSEMARY NEEDLES

½ TEASPOON LAVENDER FLOWERS

½ TEASPOON CILANTRO LEAVES

½-INCH GINGER ROOT

2 CUPS WATER

Bring water to a boil, then add herbs. Remove from heat, cover, and steep for twenty to thirty minutes. Strain and, if desired, add sweetener of choice. Compost or discard herbs. Drink at desired temperature over the course of two hours.

### ESSENTIAL OIL: *Ear Oil Poultice*

These essential oils are known to open the blood vessels and increase circulation to the ears. Try this recipe daily for one week to get the blood pumping through the ears and increase hearing abilities.

6 DROPS CAJEPUT OIL

6 DROPS TEA TREE OIL

1 LINEN SQUARE

Pour the drops of oil onto the linen. Lay on the opposite side of the ear with the hearing loss—your ear should be facing upward for treatment. Place the linen on the ear and rest for ten to twenty minutes. Repeat on opposite ear if needed. Complete entire process daily for one week. Do not get any of the oil directly into the ear canal.

### HOME REMEDY: *Old-Time Salt Poultice*

All over the world, people have used salt poultices to draw any moisture out of the ear canal and warm the ear. Never place salt directly in the ear. Any type of salt may be used, but we always use kosher salt, as it is larger and does not get wet as easily or spill from the cloth.

2 TABLESPOONS KOSHER SALT

1 LARGE LINEN SQUARE

Place the salt into the middle of the cloth. Draw up the edges and tie tightly in the middle, making a salt bag. Lie with the ear to be treated facing upward. Place the salt poultice on the ear. Rest for twenty minutes, allowing time for the salt to draw any moisture out of the ear. Repeat the process up to three times daily for one week. You may reuse the salt bag until moisture forms on the outside of the bag, usually up to a week.

• • • •

# Heartburn (Acid Indigestion)

Heartburn and acid indigestion are uncomfortable, persistent, and tend to linger all day and night. Heartburn, or acid indigestion, can be a symptom of more serious diseases, so a professional diagnosis is recommended. There are a thousand remedies for aiding oneself of typical heartburn and indigestion symptoms. These are my favorite recipes from around the world.

### AYURVEDA: *Pitta Heartburn Reducer*

It is believed in Ayurvedic practices that the imbalance of the pitta dosha is responsible for heartburn, GERD, acid reflux, and many other digestive ailments. Below are Ayurvedic tips to reduce pitta and get the stomach back to its healthy state.

- Add turmeric to meals as often as possible. Other herbs to add include basil, fennel seeds, coriander, cloves, and mint. These herbs and spices help to soothe the stomach and esophagus.

- Drink a glass of milk or coconut milk at the onset of the heartburn.

- Avoid fried foods, alcohol, and acidic foods such as oranges, pickles, vinegar, and other citruses.

- Eat a healthy breakfast. An empty stomach is a vessel filling with acid. Eat kitchari (lentils and rice) when possible, as it soothes the stomach and repels acid.

- Try to avoid stress. Meditate and walk in nature to reduce acid in the stomach.

### HERB: *Indigestion Infusion*

Herbs have been used for centuries to reduce heartburn and bring relief to the esophagus, stomach, and digestive tract. Herbs such as marshmallow root, basil, German chamomile, and licorice root, as well as the herbs listed below, have been used for thousands of years to aid in the termination of heartburn.

2 TABLESPOONS ANGELICA

3 TABLESPOONS PEPPERMINT

3 TABLESPOONS LEMON BALM

1 PINT WATER

Place the herbs into a pan with the pint of water. Cook on very low heat for one hour until liquid is reduced by half. Turn off heat, cover, and steep between one and three hours. Strain and, if desired, add sweetener of choice. Compost or discard herbs. Reserve the liquid in a jar with a tight-fitting lid. Sip a spoonful of the infusion once every thirty minutes to an hour. Store remainder in refrigerator for up to three days.

## ESSENTIAL OIL: *Heartburn and Indigestion Soother*

Essential oils contain anti-inflammatory, antispasmodic, antiemetic, and digestive healing properties to reduce acid, soothe the digestive tract, and bring relief to heartburn sufferers.

5 DROPS PEPPERMINT OIL

3 DROPS FRANKINCENSE OIL

3 DROPS CARDAMOM OIL

2 DROPS BASIL OIL

1 OUNCE CARRIER OIL (SUCH AS JOJOBA, SESAME, GRAPESEED, OR YOUR PREFERENCE)

4 DROPS VITAMIN E OIL

Mix the ingredients in a small glass container and apply lightly to the area desired, such as chest, abdomen, and throat. Keep essential oil mixture away from open wounds, mucus membranes, genitals, eyes, and sensitive areas. Repeat application as needed, usually two to three times daily. Store unused portion in a glass jar with a tight-fitting lid, label it, and keep it in a cool, dark area for up to six months.

## HOME REMEDY: *Natural Indigestion Remedies*

Studies and experience have proven that several simple methods can be incorporated into your lifestyle to reduce the chances of experiencing acid reflux, heartburn, and a multitude of digestive issues. These include, but are not limited to, the following tips and hints:

- Sleep on your left side.

- Drink chamomile tea after meals.

- Eat non-spicy, non-greasy foods. Control weight gain with healthy eating of fresh produce and non-prepackaged foods.

- Take a walk or perform mild exercise after each meal.

· · · ·
# HEAT EXHAUSTION

Heat exhaustion results from countless sources, but mainly from extended exposure to heat or sun. Ensure that the person is not suffering from heat stroke, as this can be fatal and requires immediate medical attention. Essential oils, herbs, Ayurveda, and natural remedies have been used for centuries to assist someone suffering from heat exhaustion.

## AYURVEDA: *Cool Onion Wonder*

Ayurvedic practitioners grab an onion if they are suffering from heat exhaustion. You can either rub the onion juice directly on the neck and behind the ears or you can bake the onion and consume it. This onion paste is the go-to treatment for heat exhaustion in India. The onion and cumin are believed to draw out the heat.

1 SMALL ONION

1 PIECE TINFOIL

½ TEASPOON CUMIN SEEDS, GROUND OR POWDERED

Peel the onion and wrap in the tinfoil. Bake the onion at 350 degrees until tender, twenty to thirty minutes. Slightly cool the onion and mash into a paste. Grind the cumin seeds into powder form or use ground cumin and mix the cumin powder into the mashed onion. Spread one-fourth of the cooled paste onto the person's chest, forehead, and behind the ears. Leave on for twenty minutes and wipe off with a wet cloth. Store remainder of onion in a container with a tight-fitting lid for up to forty-eight hours. Repeat process as needed.

## HERB: *Cool Me Down Tea*

These herbs have been used for years to reduce heat and bring cooling to the body.

**1 TEASPOON CORIANDER**

**1 TEASPOON MINT LEAVES**

**1 CUP WATER**

Place the herbs into boiling water. Remove from heat, cover, and steep for six to eight minutes. Strain and, if desired, add sweetener of choice. Compost or discard herbs.

## ESSENTIAL OIL: *Quick Cooling Oil Relief*

One of the quickest ways to bring down the body's temperature is to apply peppermint oil. This remedy has been used for ages. Peppermint has cooling agents that work to bring the temperature back under control.

**2 DROPS PEPPERMINT OIL**

Place the peppermint oil onto the fingertip and rub one drop of the oil behind each ear. Follow up by placing a cool cloth on the forehead and allowing the person room to breathe and cool down. Do not apply essential oils to mucus membranes.

## HOME REMEDY: *Body Cooling*

Many home remedies work wonders for ridding the body of heat and cooling us down. When out in the heat for too long, use common sense and don't overdo it. If feeling nauseous, dizzy, or weak, sit in the shade. Here are a few easy-to-apply remedies to help you get back on your feet and back to enjoying your surroundings.

- Loosen the clothing and allow air to circulate.

- Drink water slowly and continue to drink it until the body is back to normal. Energy drinks, coconut water, and cool herbal teas will all work to bring the body temperature back to normal.

- Get out of the sun and into the shade. If possible, use a fan to circulate cooler air.

- Place cool cloths on the forehead and behind the neck to bring body temperature down.

- Swallow a spoonful of ½ teaspoon honey mixed with ½ teaspoon apple cider vinegar. These work like Gatorade in restoring electrolytes to the body.

- Take a bath in cool water. Ensure the person is feeling better before they get into tepid water. If the person is losing consciousness, then do not give them a bath but transport them immediately to an emergency room.

· · · ·

# HEMORRHOIDS

Hemorrhoids can lead to very serious complications, surgery, and months of debilitation. Ayurveda, home remedies, essential oils, and herbs work with therapeutic properties to reduce the swelling and inflammation of the veins in the anal region. Before pharmacies and drugstores, hemorrhoids were dealt with in a more natural way. I have gathered a few of these old recipes for you to replicate for relief.

### AYURVEDA: *Witch Hazel Pad*

Witch hazel has been used for centuries to heal hemorrhoids. This is the number one hemorrhoid treatment in India. It is pain-relieving, cooling, and also relieves the itching.

**1 TABLESPOON WITCH HAZEL**

**1 GAUZE OR LINEN SQUARE**

Soak the gauze or linen square with the witch hazel. Apply to hemorrhoid and leave in place inside of underwear. Leave on for as long as comfortable. Reapply as needed.

## HERB: *Comfortable Comfrey*

Comfrey has been used for generations to ease the discomfort of hemorrhoids. This rub is easy to make and works well on most people.

**1 TABLESPOON COMFREY ROOT POWDER**

**½ OUNCE CARRIER OIL (SUCH AS JOJOBA, SESAME, GRAPESEED, OR YOUR PREFERENCE)**

**1 GAUZE OR LINEN SQUARE**

In a small container with a lid, mix the herb and the carrier oil with a whisk. Soak the gauze or linen square with the herbal oil. Apply to hemorrhoid and leave in place inside of underwear. Leave on for as long as comfortable. Reapply as needed. Store remainder at room temperature for up to forty-eight hours.

## ESSENTIAL OIL: *Itch-Relieving Bath*

This bath contains ingredients that reduce the inflammation, itch, and pain associated with hemorrhoids. This bath feels so good and relieves much of the suffering.

**8 DROPS HELICHRYSUM OIL**

**8 DROPS LAVENDER OIL**

**8 DROPS YARROW OIL**

**¼ CUP WITCH HAZEL**

**1 TABLESPOON MILK (OPTIONAL)**

As you begin to fill the tub with water, pour the essential oils and witch hazel into the running water. Run a warm, not hot, bath. Water that is too hot will cause the essential oils to dissipate.If you add milk to the water, it will prevent the oil from floating on top of the water and sticking to your skin. Soak in the water as long as you are comfortable.

## HOME REMEDY: *Vein Shrinker Drink*

The vinegar works to shrink the capillaries, the honey is an anti-inflammatory, and the cayenne pepper works to end the hemorrhoids.

½ CUP HONEY

½ CUP APPLE CIDER VINEGAR

1 CUP WATER

1 CAYENNE PEPPER, CHOPPED

Mix all of the ingredients together in a mason jar and shake well. Strain and discard pepper, reserving liquid. Before or after each meal, take a tablespoon of the well-mixed blend. Store remainder in a jar with a tight-fitting lid in the refrigerator. Discard after three days. Shake or stir well before each usage.

• • • •

# HICCUPS

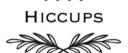

Hiccups are annoying, embarrassing, and have spawned a thousand remedies. A catch in the diaphragm is the culprit. Usually time alone can end the hiccups, but here are a few recipes and tips to get rid of them.

## AYURVEDA: *Ayurvedic Hiccup Destroyer*

In Ayurvedic treatments of hiccups, this remedy is the most often used. Take slowly and enjoy the textures as you put an end to those hiccups.

1 TEASPOON HONEY

¼ TEASPOON GROUND GINGER

Mix the ingredients into a spoon. Slowly drink the ingredients. The change in your swallowing and breathing patterns should relax the esophagus and end those hiccups.

## HERB: *Hiccup Tea*

This sweet-tasting tea has been used worldwide to end hiccups. Add a sweetener of choice to make this tea into a delightful desert!

**1 CUP WATER**

**1 TEASPOON GROUND CARDAMOM SEEDS**

Bring water to a boil, then add seeds. Remove from heat, cover, and steep for six minutes. Strain and, if desired, add sweetener of choice.

## ESSENTIAL OIL: *Breathe the Air*

The essential oils in this diffuser blend work together to put an end to your hiccups and relax those throat muscles.

**5 DROPS MANDARIN OIL**

**3 DROPS SANDALWOOD OIL**

**3 DROPS DILL OIL**

**WATER**

Add oils and water to diffuser and run as desired.

## HOME REMEDY: *Hiccup Home Remedies*

Surely in your lifetime you have tried a couple of these home remedies and tips from various cultures. Some of them are fun and some of them are yucky, but all of them have worked for one person or another. The changes in breathing patterns, swallowing, and muscle movement in all of the tips below work to get that diaphragm back to normal.

- Slowly eat a spoonful of sugar, honey, or peanut butter.
- BOO! Scare the person with the hiccups.
  A sudden fright is supposed to end them.
- Slowly lick ¼ teaspoon hot sauce.
- A spoonful of vinegar is reported to end hiccups quickly.
- Hold your breath for as long as you can. This change
  in breathing patterns should do the trick.
- Breathe into a paper bag for a minute.

- Hang your head upside down. Drink a glass of water while in this position.

- Drink a glass of water through a small straw.

- Chew a small piece of ginger and swallow.

# HIGH BLOOD PRESSURE

High blood pressure is a condition in which the blood pressure in the arteries is elevated. Medication is available to regulate the blood pressure through your doctor. High blood pressure is nothing to ignore. It can cause serious complications. Diet and exercise play a huge role in regulating blood pressure. Professional medical care and treatment is essential. Essential oils, herbs, home remedies, and Ayurvedic treatments can often relax a person and assist them with reducing their blood pressure. Ensure through a physician that the treatments will not interfere with current medications.

## AYURVEDA: *Pressure Reducer*

Flaxseed has been known to lower blood pressure and reduce other issues, according to Ayurvedic medicine. This blend works wonders to get the blood pumping properly and has been used in the East for thousands of years.

**1 TEASPOON GROUND FLAXSEED**

**½ CUP COCONUT WATER**

Chew the flaxseed well and swallow, then follow with the coconut water. This blend is refreshing and will have you feeling better in minutes.

## HERB: *Lowering Syrup*

Berries, lemons, and cinnamon have been used for centuries to lower blood pressure. A tablespoonful of this syrup every morning works throughout the day to reduce blood pressure, not to mention that it tastes like heaven!

**2 CUPS WATER**

**3 TABLESPOONS BLUEBERRIES**

**3 TABLESPOONS ELDERBERRIES**

**½ TEASPOON CINNAMON**

**½ CUP HONEY**

**1 TEASPOON LEMON JUICE**

Pour water in a pan and bring to a boil. Add the berries and reduce heat to low. Cover and heat until almost half the water is gone. Remove from heat; leave covered and steep for one hour. Strain, then add cinnamon, honey, and lemon juice while liquid is still hot and stir. Add more honey until it reaches desired thickness. Cool and place in bottle. Store in refrigerator for up to one week.

## ESSENTIAL OIL: *Anxiety Powder*

Ridding oneself of anxiety, fear, and stress is one of the best ways to reduce blood pressure. This powder contains essential oils that have been scientifically proven to reduce blood pressure. This blend will have you falling asleep quickly, without worry and stress.

**5 DROPS FRENCH LAVENDER OIL**

**8 DROPS FRANKINCENSE OIL**

**3 DROPS CASSIA OIL**

**5 DROPS VITAMIN E OIL**

**1 CUP CORNSTARCH**

Place the ingredients into a mason jar, stirring well. Carefully poke holes into the lid and use this as a shaker to dispense the ingredients into pillowcases or under sheets as needed. You can get a piece of plastic wrap and place it over the jar and under the lid to keep powder from spilling out when not in use. Label and store in a cool, dark, dry area for up to three months.

## HOME REMEDY: *Daily Pressure Salad*

Anyone with high blood pressure should watch their diet very closely. This recipe is delicious and full of blood pressure–reducing herbs, vegetables, and ingredients. Try to eat this a couple of times a week, especially on very stressful days.

2 CUPS SPINACH LEAVES

½ CUP CUBED MELON

2 TABLESPOONS FRESH BASIL LEAVES

2 TABLESPOONS FRESH BERRIES

2 TABLESPOONS OLIVE OIL

¼ TEASPOON LEMON JUICE

1 TEASPOON HONEY

½ TEASPOON GARLIC, MINCED

½ TEASPOON MINCED GINGER

Mix the spinach, melon, basil, and berries in a large bowl. In a small container, combine the oil, lemon, honey, garlic, and ginger until well blended. Pour the dressing onto the salad and mix lightly. Store remainder in the refrigerator for up to twenty-four hours.

• • • •

# HIVES

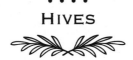

Hives are an allergic reaction causing raised red welts on the skin. People can get hives repeatedly without knowing what it is causing this reaction. The best way to address this is to write down everything you eat or use on your body each time you have a reaction. Take the journaling about your hives to a diagnostician if you are having trouble finding the answer yourself. Ayurveda, herbs, essential oils, and home remedies abound for ridding oneself of hives.

### AYURVEDA: *Hive Paste*

In Ayurvedic teachings turmeric is quite the little miracle. This anti-inflammatory and cicatrisant-loaded ingredient will work wonders on your hives, reducing itching, swelling, and overall appearance.

1 TABLESPOON TURMERIC

2 TABLESPOONS MILK

½ TEASPOON GROUND GINGER

Combine the ingredients together well. Using fingers, smear the paste onto the hive areas and allow to air-dry. If you must go out, you may tape some gauze over the area loosely. Turmeric will stain furniture and clothing, so use old clothing and sit on a sheet or towel to protect the furniture. Once you feel the paste is flaking off or no longer effective, rinse with tepid water. Reapply as needed.

## HERB: *Hive Tea*

These herbs work from the inside out to bring you relief from your hives. Drink two to three cups a day until the hives are gone.

> 1 CUP WATER
>
> 1 TEASPOON MINT LEAVES
>
> 1 TEASPOON GRATED GINGER
>
> JUICE FROM ½ LEMON

Bring water to a boil, then add herbs. Remove from heat, cover, and steep for six to eight minutes. Strain. Add lemon juice and, if desired, sweetener of choice. Compost or discard herbs.

## ESSENTIAL OIL: *Hive Oil Spray*

These essential oils work well together to bring that itching under control, reduce swelling, and give you instant relief. The anti-inflammatory, anti-itch, antiallergenic, antibiotic, analgesic, and astringent properties in these oils are perfect for hives.

> 8 DROPS MYRRH OIL
>
> 7 DROPS FRANKINCENSE OIL
>
> 5 DROPS TEA TREE OIL
>
> 5 DROPS PEPPERMINT OIL
>
> 5 DROPS VITAMIN E OIL
>
> 1 TEASPOON WITCH HAZEL
>
> 2 OUNCES WATER

Combine the ingredients into a spray bottle and shake well. Lightly spray the area of the body covered with hives and allow to air-dry. Do not spray into eyes, mouth, genitals, open wounds, or mucus membranes. Shake well before each use. Store in a cool, dark area for up to three months.

### HOME REMEDY: *Hive Bath Soak*

These soothing ingredients work together to bring you instant relief.

**½ CUP OATMEAL**

**¼ CUP BAKING SODA**

Once the bathwater has run, put the ingredients into a square of cloth and tie into a ball. Rub the ball over the hive-affected body area. Soak in tub for twenty minutes or until water is no longer comfortable.

• • • •

# HORMONE IMBALANCE

There are many essential oils, herbs, Ayurvedic practices, and home remedies that contain natural hormones which can create a balance without using artificial hormones. Hormone-balancing recipes utilizing natural ingredients are very beneficial during an already tumultuous time.

### AYURVEDA: *Hormone Decoction*

Ashwagandha root is called the ginseng of India. Its powerful properties give energy to you as well as natural hormone balancing and an overall tonic. This decoction is great to have on hand when fatigue and mental clarity are at a low.

**½-INCH Ashwagandha ROOT, GRATED**

**2 CUPS WATER**

**1 TEASPOON HONEY**

Add the grated root to boiling water and simmer for twenty minutes. Let sit in hot water for ten more minutes after removing from stove. Strain, cool, add honey, and drink throughout the day.

## HERB: *Herbal Hormone Salve*

Apply this salve daily to your body to reduce fatigue, level out hormones, calm an overanxious mind, and bring a sense of normalcy to your life. Menopause, having a baby, and life stressors can cause our hormones to plummet or spiral out of control. The natural hormone balancers in this recipe and the ease of applying to your body make this salve an ideal alternative treatment to chemicals and pharmaceuticals.

> ¼ OUNCE HOLY BASIL LEAVES
>
> ¼ OUNCE RASPBERRY LEAVES
>
> ¼ OUNCE CALENDULA FLOWERS
>
> ¼ OUNCE ST. JOHN'S WORT
>
> 1½ CUPS CARRIER OIL (SUCH AS JOJOBA, SESAME, GRAPESEED, OR YOUR PREFERENCE)
>
> 1–1½ OUNCES BEESWAX
>
> ½ TEASPOON GROUND TURMERIC
>
> 6 DROPS VITAMIN E OIL

Pack the herbs into the carrier oil and cook on low on stovetop for an hour and a half. Strain through cheesecloth into a glass bowl and add beeswax, stirring until beeswax is melted. Add turmeric and vitamin E and stir. Pour a drop of the mixture onto the counter. Run your finger through the drop after a few seconds of cooling—if it is too thick, add a little oil; if it is too thin, add a little more beeswax. Once you are happy with the consistency, pour into a jar and label. Cool before applying to skin. Apply to desired area by rubbing or massaging into the skin. Store in a cool, dark area for up to one year.

## ESSENTIAL OIL: *Hormone Salt Bath*

This salt bath contains essential oils that are essential to balancing your hormones. Therapeutic properties work to calm you, cool your body, reduce bloating, and bring a sense of peace. These jars make attractive, inexpensive, and healing gifts!

10 DROPS BORAGE OIL

10 DROPS BERGAMOT OIL

10 DROPS NEROLI OIL

2 TABLESPOONS CARRIER OIL (SUCH AS JOJOBA, SESAME, GRAPESEED, OR YOUR PREFERENCE)

3 CUPS SALT (PINK HIMALAYAN, SEA, EPSOM, OR YOUR PREFERENCE)

1 TABLESPOON MILK (OPTIONAL)

Add the essential oils and carrier oil to salt. Stir until essential oil and salt mixture are well blended. Cover tightly. Leave mixture in a dark area for twenty-four hours, then stir mixture again. Run the bathwater, but not so hot as to ruin the oils. Add a half cup of the bath salt mixture to bathwater. If you add milk to the water, it will prevent the oil from floating on top of the water and sticking to your skin. Store remainder in a glass jar with a tight-fitting lid in a cool, dark area for up to three months.

## HOME REMEDY: *Daily Hormone Salad*

This salad contains many of the foods recommended to balance hormones. Try these foods in other recipes and bring your mind, body, and spirit back under your own control.

1 CUP BROCCOLI, CHOPPED

1 AVOCADO, DICED

1 SMALL TOMATO, DICED

1 TABLESPOON WALNUTS, CHOPPED

½ TEASPOON FLAXSEED OR CHIA SEEDS

½ TEASPOON COCONUT OIL

¼ TEASPOON LEMON JUICE

1 DASH HOT SAUCE

Combine all of the vegetables and seeds into a bowl and stir well. In another container whisk together the coconut oil, lemon juice, and hot sauce. Stir into salad and add salt and pepper to taste. Eat with crackers, cheese, or vegetable sticks.

· · · ·

# HOT FLASHES

Once a woman reaches a certain point in her life, internal temperature regulators go a little haywire. This causes intense heat flashes within the body, and little can be done to cool you down. Night sweats, hot flashes, and mood swings are all a normal part of this cycle. Natural healing remedies—including Ayurvedic treatments, herbal treatments, and usage of essential oils and herbs—can all play a part in helping us to reduce hot flashes and regulate the body temperature.

### AYURVEDA: *Ayurvedic Cooling Massage*

A scalp massage is one of the quickest ways of cooling or heating the body, depending on what herb or treatment you apply. Brahmi is well known for its cooling properties. This massage is great for cooling the body down for several hours. Try to get it mainly on your scalp, not in your hair.

**1 TEASPOON BRAHMI OIL**

Dip your fingertips into the oil and gently massage the scalp all over the head. This oil can also be used in your conditioner, but you will have to shake the bottle very well before each usage. Once the oil is on your scalp, be sure to use a protective covering on your pillowcase, as the oil will stain material. In the morning, wash and rinse hair as usual.

### HERB: *Hot Flash Tincture*

The cooling, heat-relieving effects of this tincture have been used for thousands of years by women suffering through hot flashes. Take a teaspoon in a shot glass of juice when you feel a hot flash coming on to stop it in its tracks.

**½ CUP CHICKWEED**

**½ CUP ST. JOHN'S WORT**

**1 PINT HIGH PROOF VODKA**

Place herbs in a pint jar until it's half full with dried herbs or two-thirds full with fresh herbs, and cover with a high proof vodka, about an inch from the top of the jar. Cover tightly and place in a cool, dark location. Shake vigorously every day for two weeks, then let it set without shaking for one month. Strain, bottle, and label, adding the date you decanted it (strained the herb). Use a half to one dropperful in tea, water, or other liquid. You can take it straight, though the taste is very strong. Tinctures made with alcohol will last up to three years if kept in a cool, dark place.

## ESSENTIAL OIL: *Hot Flash Spray*

Mints are naturally cooling. This spray is such a relief to an intensely over-heated body. Just spray it on your face, chest, and in the air to cool down the body instantly. I like to keep a little bottle of this by my bedside. When a hot flash wakes me up in the middle of the night, I just throw off the covers and give a spray or two of this high in the air over my body. The mist settles on my body and by the time it air-dries, my hot flash is gone.

**20 DROPS SPEARMINT OIL**

**1 TEASPOON WITCH HAZEL**

**1 OUNCE WATER**

Add all ingredients to a dark-colored spray bottle. Shake bottle and spray onto area desired during hot flash. Do not spray into open wounds, genitals, eyes, or mucus membranes. Store in a cool, dark area for up to three months. Shake well before each use to combine the ingredients.

## HOME REMEDY: *Home Remedies for Hot Flashes*

There have been many remedies passed down from mother to daughter throughout the ages on how to deal with hot flashes. Try a few of these tips that not only help to keep the body finely tuned to dispel heat, but they also bring an overall wellness.

- Stay hydrated. Drink plenty of water throughout the day and keep a glass by your bedside at night.
- Don't smoke.
- Keep a well-balanced, lowfat, high fiber diet. Try to eat plenty of vegetables.

- Sleep on cotton sheets. Synthetic blends tend to induce sweating and hot flashes.

- Wear cotton underwear and pajamas (maybe not as sexy as silk, but much more cooling).

- Exercise daily. Moderate bursts of high intensity followed by soothing stretches seem to work the best at reducing hot flashes.

- No caffeine, no spicy food, and no sugar or alcohol.

- Meditate daily, even if you only have five minutes. Deep breathing and thinking pleasant thoughts can work wonders in reducing stress. Stress is a catapult for hot flashes.

- Drink water with lemon in it. Lemon is very detoxifying and will help to rid your body of the thousands of poisons that can collect in our bodies daily.

- Sleep with an air conditioner or a fan. Cooling the room around you will help in cooling your insides, too.

- Stay out of the sun and get in the shade as much as possible. Sun brings on hot flashes quickly. Being outdoors is very important to your overall well-being, so try to walk in shady areas.

- Wear loose clothing as much as possible. Light linen and cotton clothing will help the air to circulate between you and your clothes.

• • • •

## IMMUNODEFICIENCY DISORDER

Having an immune deficiency opens you up to every disease in the world. Our immune system is like a bunch of tiny soldiers who battle viruses, bacteria, and disease daily as they invade our body. Building up our immunity army is paramount to good health. Illness, heredity, diet, environmental factors, and living conditions all affect our immunity and can cause immunodeficiency disorder. These recipes have been used for a long time to help us fight against the tiny disease carriers that surround us. Try some and see if you don't have a healthier and happier life.

## AYURVEDA: *Immunity Tips*

For thousands of years, people have used the following practices to strengthen their immune systems, and scientific evidence shows that they do work. Try to incorporate these Ayurvedic remedies into your daily life to give your health the edge you need.

- Alternate nostril breathing. Sitting cross-legged on the floor, breathe through your right nostril for five breaths while covering your left nostril with your left thumb. Then breathe through your left nostril for five breaths while covering your right nostril with your right thumb. Continue this peaceful, healing ritual for five minutes twice daily.

- Turmeric is a vitamin-rich, antioxidant-laden spice that should be added to as many meals as you can incorporate it into.

- Completing a series of slow, stretching yoga moves every day has been proven to boost the immune system and lower incidences of illness among practitioners.

- Try meditating five minutes a day and work your way up to twenty minutes daily. Sit in a peaceful, quiet place and just let your mind wander to where it will. Concentrate on your breathing, slowly in and out. Do not force anything; just let your mind go. Meditation has improved the health of millions of people.

## HERB: *Immunity Tea*

These herbs are all antioxidants that fight invaders to the body, and they can strengthen our immunity system.

1 CUP WATER

1 TEASPOON ECHINACEA FLOWERS

1 TEASPOON GRATED GINGER

1 TEASPOON CHAMOMILE FLOWERS

1 TEASPOON HONEY (OPTIONAL)

Bring water to a boil, then add herbs. Remove from heat, cover, and steep for six to eight minutes. Strain and compost or discard herbs. If desired, add honey or sweetener of choice. Drink two or three cups weekly to keep immune system in great working order.

## ESSENTIAL OIL: *Immunity Diffuser*

These essential oils are full of immune boosting properties. Fill this diffuser and give everyone in your household or office a fighting chance against germs and bacteria.

**5** DROPS FRANKINCENSE OIL

**5** DROPS GRAPEFRUIT OIL

**4** DROPS TEA TREE OIL

WATER

Add oils and water to diffuser and run as desired.

## HOME REMEDY: *Immunity Builder*

These common-sense remedies work to rid the body of toxins, boost immunity, restore depleted vitamins and minerals, and give a person the benefits of having a healthier lifestyle. As many of these tips as possible should be practiced daily.

- A deep tissue massage not only feels wonderful, but it rids the body of deeply buried toxins, brings a sense of calm, and rids the body and mind of any anxiety.

- Wash your hands. This kindergarten practice was developed for a reason. If your hands are continually spreading illness to you and others, your body will use all of your immunity resources fighting something that could have been destroyed by soap and water.

- Consume citrus fruits, orange vegetables, leafy green vegetables, flaxseed, chia seeds, garlic, onions, lightly cooked meals, and cranberry juice. Add herbal teas to your daily diet such as green tea, chamomile tea, ginseng tea, echinacea tea, and ginger tea.

- Take a probiotic daily to help your digestive tract heal and fight bacteria as it should.

- The best vitamins to help build an immune system are vitamin A, vitamin B6, vitamin E, and zinc.

- If possible, avoid alcohol, red meat, sugar, and heavy, overcooked meals.

- Get plenty of exercise daily. Walk in nature. Swim or do yoga, cardio, or any type of exercise that helps you to breathe in and out and get the best benefits from oxygen.

• • • •

# IMPETIGO

Impetigo is a highly contagious infection of the skin caused by bacteria spreading from one person to another. It causes red raised sores on the skin that don't heal well. For thousands of years, herbs, medicines, and essential oils that have antibacterial properties have been used to rid people, mainly children, of this painful and scarring condition. Your doctor can prescribe medicines that are also very effective at healing the infection.

## AYURVEDA: *Impetigo Oil*

This centuries-old Ayurvedic recipe is loaded with antibacterial properties to promote healing and kill bacteria. Garlic is one of the most powerful antibacterial agents on earth. Use antibiotic cream alternately with this oil.

**1 TABLESPOON SESAME OIL**

**1 CLOVE GARLIC, MINCED**

**¼ TEASPOON TURMERIC POWDER**

Heat oil on low in a small pan. Add the minced garlic and simmer on low for two to three minutes. Remove from heat and carefully strain the oil. Discard the garlic. Add the turmeric powder and stir. Once cooled, apply to the wound. Cover with gauze. Leave on for several hours or overnight. Store remainder in a container with a lid for up to twenty-four hours at room temperature. Apply two to three times daily.

## HERB: *Impetigo Herbal Paste*

This easy herbal remedy is very effective in most cases. The antibacterial properties of goldenseal, applied several times daily, work wonders in fighting bacterial infections.

**1 TEASPOON GOLDENSEAL POWDER**

**1–2 TEASPOONS WATER**

Combine the ingredients into a paste. Apply to affected area and cover with gauze. Leave on overnight or for several hours. Reapply until wound is crusted over and looks dry. Store remainder of ingredients in a covered container and use within twenty-four hours.

## ESSENTIAL OIL: *Impetigo Gauze*

This remedy includes powerful antibacterial components to end the infection and bring instant relief.

**2 DROPS TEA TREE OIL**

**2 DROPS HELICHRYSUM OIL**

**2 DROPS MYRRH OIL**

**¼ TEASPOON CARRIER OIL (SUCH AS JOJOBA, SESAME, GRAPESEED, OR YOUR PREFERENCE)**

Apply mixture of oils to a piece of gauze. Secure gauze to site of impetigo. Leave on for several hours or overnight. Cover any remaining mixture and use within forty-eight hours. Store at room temperature.

## HOME REMEDY: *Vinegar Wash Remedy*

This ancient home remedy uses vinegar as the antibacterial agent. Remember that impetigo is very highly contagious, and caution should be applied when treating this condition. All clothing, towels, etc., should be washed separately from the general laundry. Keep wound clean at all times.

**2 TABLESPOONS WHITE VINEGAR**

**2 CUPS WATER**

Combine ingredients into a bowl. Use a cloth or a cotton ball to apply the wash to the clean wound. Cover with light gauze or linen. Repeat procedure several times daily until wound is crusted over and appears dry. Store any remainder at room temperature and use within forty-eight hours.

• • • •

# INFECTION

Infections can be deadly if left untreated. Minor infections can be easily treated by home remedies, but infections that cause fever, fatigue, or a host of other symptoms should be treated by medical professionals. In the event that you have a minor infection, try some of these infection-fighting treatments from around the world. If infection spreads, causes fever, or is painful, seek medical attention.

### AYURVEDA: *Sun Gazing*

I find this treatment fascinating. NASA, scientists, and practitioners from all over the world study this phenomenon, and there have been numerous amounts of research over the beneficial effects of sun gazing on the body. Infection cases have definitely been documented to have been healed many times by sun gazing.

One must be barefoot and connected directly to the earth to sun gaze. Sit comfortably and wear comfortable clothing. The time is very important. It must be within thirty minutes of sunrise or sunset. Gazing at the sun any other time of the day will damage the optic nerves and the retinas. At sunrise or sunset, sit before the sun and gaze at it while either chanting, praying, meditating, or thinking of nothing except pleasant thoughts. Start out with ten or twenty seconds the first day. Increase by ten or twenty seconds daily until you can gaze at the sun for thirty minutes. It will take several months to reach this stage. The sun is said to be one of the most powerful healing agents known to humankind.

## HERB: *Respiratory Infection Syrup*

Elderberries have powerful antibacterial and anti-infective properties. This recipe has been used for generations to bring comfort and ease to people with respiratory, head, and throat infections.

   1 CUP ELDERBERRIES

   3 CUPS WATER

   4 TABLESPOONS LEMON JUICE

   3 TABLESPOONS HONEY

Bring water to a boil. Add elderberries and reduce heat to low. Cover and heat until almost half the water is gone. Remove from heat, leave covered, and steep for one hour. Strain liquid and add lemon juice and honey while liquid is still hot; stir. You may add more honey until it reaches desired thickness. Cool and place in bottle. Standard dosage is one tablespoon for adults and one teaspoon for children as needed. Store in refrigerator for up to one month.

## ESSENTIAL OIL: *Infection Oil Foot Rub*

The soles of the feet are the quickest carriers of essential oils to every cell in the body. When suffering from an infection inside of the body, try using this foot rub and you will be delivering anti-infective properties quickly to where they are needed.

   10 DROPS TEA TREE OIL

   10 DROP OREGANO OIL

   1 OUNCE CARRIER OIL (SUCH AS JOJOBA, SESAME, GRAPESEED, OR YOUR PREFERENCE)

   4 DROPS VITAMIN E OIL

Mix the ingredients in a small glass container and apply lightly to the soles of feet. Prevent slipping and hurting yourself by sitting with your feet up for fifteen minutes or wearing slippers after applying. Keep essential oil mixture away from open wounds, mucus membranes, genitals, eyes, and sensitive areas. Repeat application as needed, usually two to three times daily. Store unused portion in a glass jar with a tight-fitting lid, label it, and keep it in a cool, dark area for up to six months.

## HOME REMEDY: *Infection Treatments*

Long before there were antibiotics and drugstores, people had to find ways to fight infections in order for the species to survive. In the course of our lives, we have many minor infections of the skin, lungs, stomach, etc. Use some of these techniques the next time you have a minor infection.

- Don't make the water so hot as to be scalding, but the steam from a regular hot shower can help protect your lungs against infections.

- Drink a cup of water with some apple cider vinegar. Antibiotic and anti-infective properties in vinegar will help to heal that infection.

- Your body uses a lot of energy fighting infections. Adequate rest and sleep will allow your body to use your energy for the fight.

- Drink juices and water and eat a healthy vegetable and fruit diet. Do not eat heavy, spicy, rich foods during times of infection.

- Drink plenty of herbal teas. Herbs contain powerful infection-fighting properties. Add lemon to aid in the detox of germs.

- Take plenty of vitamin C and drink orange juice and other citrus drinks.

- Rest outside if it is a nice day. Nature plays an important part in helping us to achieve our healthiest defenses against infection by lowering our stress and allowing our immune system to fight other battles.

- Take ginger, turmeric, and garlic as often as possible in meals, drinks, poultices, and other avenues. These foods have some of the most powerful antibiotics on earth.

• • • •

# INFLAMMATION

Inflammation comes in many forms for many reasons. Redness, swelling, and pain can flare up inside or outside of our bodies. People have used herbs, oils, ancient methods, and home remedies to reduce inflammation throughout history. If inflammation is a result of infection, seek medical attention at once.

### AYURVEDA: *Turmeric Milk*

This paste can be kept in the refrigerator for a week. Turmeric is one of the most natural anti-inflammatory agents on earth. Add a teaspoon of this paste mixture to a cup of warm milk as often as you like and drink. The benefits are amazing: pain will be reduced, inflammation will dissipate, and you will feel like a million bucks.

**4 TABLESPOONS TURMERIC POWDER**

**¼ CUP WATER**

Whisk together turmeric and water until a thick paste forms. Cover tightly and refrigerate. When you desire turmeric milk, just stir a teaspoon of the paste into the glass of warm milk and drink for inflammation and pain treatment. This will become one of your favorite remedies—it is for me!

### HERB: *Willow Bark Tea*

Willow bark has been used forever in treating inflammation inside of the body. With its analgesic properties, drink this tea for pain relief and to reduce swelling in the joints. Lemon and honey are also great anti-inflammatory additions to any cup of herbal tea.

**1 TEASPOON WILLOW BARK**

**1 CUP BOILING WATER**

**1 TEASPOON HONEY**

**¼ TEASPOON LEMON JUICE**

Place the willow bark into the boiling water. Remove from heat, cover, and steep for six to eight minutes. Strain and add lemon and honey. Compost or discard herbs.

## ESSENTIAL OIL: *Inflammatory Rub*

This essential oil recipe works well to reduce pain and swelling. The therapeutic properties of anti-inflammatory, antispasmodic, anti-infective, and antibacterial agents work together to bring you much-needed relief.

7 DROPS TEA TREE OIL

5 DROPS PEPPERMINT OIL

5 DROPS HELICHRYSUM OIL

2 DROPS CASSIA OIL

4 DROPS VITAMIN E OIL

1 OUNCE CARRIER OIL (SUCH AS JOJOBA, SESAME, GRAPESEED, OR YOUR PREFERENCE)

Mix the ingredients in a small glass container and apply lightly to the area desired, such as pressure points, neck, soles of feet, temples, and chest. Keep essential oil mixture away from open wounds, mucus membranes, genitals, eyes, and sensitive areas. Repeat application as needed, usually two to three times daily. Store unused portion in a glass jar with a tight-fitting lid, label it, and keep it in a cool, dark area for up to six months.

## HOME REMEDY: *Inflammatory Relief*

When your joints and muscles are inflamed due to overexertion, arthritis, or any number of complaints, try this old home remedy. It really works well to reduce swelling, inflammation, and bring instant relief.

Using two hot water bottles, alternate filling them with ice water and hot water. Using a towel or piece of linen, lay the material on the inflamed area. Lay the hot water bottle on the material and enjoy the sensation of heat. After fifteen minutes, remove the hot bottle and replace with the cold bottle. Complete this cycle two or three times daily for ultimate inflammatory relief.

• • • •

# INSECT BITES AND STINGS

Insect bites can range from minor annoyances to critical emergencies. Medical treatment should be sought for anyone who has insect bite/sting allergies or from multiple bites/stings from certain insects. For everyday bites/stings, these recipes have been used all over the world and are still relevant today. Any sting or bite that is followed by labored breathing requires a call to 911 or a trip to the emergency room.

## AYURVEDA: *Bug Treatment*

After being stung or bitten, in India and countries that practice the ancient healing of Ayurveda, honey and lemon are the go-to treatments. The anti-inflammatory and anti-infective properties of these ingredients work together to bring instant relief and healing to all types of insect bites.

**¼ TEASPOON HONEY**

**A FEW DROPS OF LEMON JUICE**

Combine the ingredients together and apply to bite or sting. You may cover with a gauze or bandage if desired. Leave on all day or night. Reapply as needed. Discard any remainder after twenty-four hours.

## HERB: *Basil Bite Paste*

I usually have basil plants growing around the house all summer. When I get stung or bitten by some little scavenger, I just grab a basil leaf, crush it up, and apply it to the bite. If you don't have any fresh basil, here is a recipe to try with dried basil.

**¼ TEASPOON BASIL LEAVES**

**¼ TEASPOON WATER**

Grind the basil leaves into powder form. Mix well with the water, forming a paste. Apply to sting or bite. You may cover with gauze or bandage if desired. Discard any remainder.

## ESSENTIAL OIL: *Bite Dabber*

Try a little dab of this on your next bite from a fire ant or any small type of insect. This recipe will bring instant relief. Various therapeutic properties work to reduce pain, itching, and swelling.

> 3 DROPS LAVENDER OIL
>
> 3 DROPS NIAOULI OIL
>
> 3 DROPS PINE OIL
>
> 3 DROPS VITAMIN E OIL
>
> ½ OUNCE CARRIER OIL (SUCH AS JOJOBA, SESAME, GRAPESEED, OR YOUR PREFERENCE)

Mix the ingredients together in a small bowl. Pour into a bottle with a tight-fitting lid and apply with finger tips or cotton swab. For ease of usage, you can put blend into a roll-on bottle. Store at room temperature for up to one year.

## HOME REMEDY: *Bites and Stings*

There are so many remedies for bug bites. This list provides us with several easy home remedies with ingredients readily available in your home. Bring relief to your itches, swelling, and irritation with these tips:

- Rub the bite with a banana peel.
- Rub the bite with a raw onion.
- Apply a fresh basil leaf to help with the itching and pain.
- Turmeric paste is a quick and easy remedy. Just combine a little turmeric with water until a paste forms and apply to the bite.

• • • •

# INSOMNIA

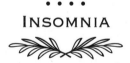

Many reasons lead to a person being unable to sleep: worry, diet, stress, noise, and more worry! Sleep studies provide evidence of various insomnia factors. There are also thousands of recipes and tips from around the world that people use to get those much-needed hours of rest.

## AYURVEDA: *Feng Shui Sleep Application*

In the Middle and Far East, it is as important how your room looks and where everything is placed as it is to have a comfortable mattress and pillow. Use these tips to help bring your bedroom up to feng shui standards and get the good night's sleep you crave:

- Your bed should be placed so that you can see the door to the bedroom. Your bed should also not have one side pushed up against the wall but should be accessible from three sides.

- It is best to have an end table on either side of the bed. Only peaceful objects should adorn the tables.

- Close all doors at bedtime. No open door or open drawers should be in the room.

- A room full of "stuff" is not conducive to rest. Put away that laundry. Pick up the things that don't need to be in there and put them somewhere else.

- Choose a painting that is happy and soothing. Don't put any depressing items in the room. Put objects in your room that bring you peace and positivity.

- When weather permits, open the windows. Fresh air not only feels good, but it is very healthy for us and can assist in the sleep process.

- Paint the walls soothing neutral colors. While bright colors may seem more appealing or modern, soft, muted colors will bring relaxation to spirit and soul.

- Soft lighting on the end tables will bring on relaxation much faster than an overhead bulb.

## HERB: *Bedtime Tea*

This ancient remedy has been used by just about everyone who has ever walked the earth, and for good reason: it works! Enjoy a cup of this tea as part of your nighttime ritual to get you relaxed enough to drift into a good night's sleep.

1 TEASPOON VALERIAN ROOT, CHOPPED

1 TEASPOON CHAMOMILE FLOWERS

1 CUP BOILING WATER

Place the herbs into the boiling water. Remove from heat, cover, and steep for eight to ten minutes. Strain and, if desired, add sweetener of choice. Compost or discard herbs.

## ESSENTIAL OIL: *Sleepy Powder*

This powder blend has sedative-inducing essential oils in the recipe. Relaxing and breathing in these aromas will help you to reduce anxiety and bring your mind and spirit to a peaceful slumber.

10 DROPS ST. JOHN'S WORT OIL

10 DROPS LEMON BALM (MELISSA) OIL

10 DROPS LAVENDER OIL

5 DROPS VITAMIN E OIL

1 CUP CORNSTARCH

Place the ingredients into a mason jar, stirring well. Carefully poke holes into the lid and use this as a shaker to dispense the ingredients into pillow-cases or under sheets as needed. You can get a piece of plastic wrap and place it over the jar and under the lid to keep powder from spilling out when not in use. Label and store in a cool, dark, dry area for up to three months.

## HOME REMEDY: *Natural Bedtime Bath Remedy*

This relaxing, aromatic bath will have you ready to hit the sack. These calming and sedative-packed oils are used worldwide for their tranquilizing properties.

8 DROPS JASMINE OIL

8 DROPS FRANKINCENSE OIL

8 DROPS VETIVER OIL

1 TABLESPOON CARRIER OIL (SUCH AS JOJOBA, SESAME, GRAPESEED, OR YOUR PREFERENCE)

1 TABLESPOON MILK (OPTIONAL)

As you begin to fill the tub with water, pour the essential oils and carrier oil into the running water. Run a warm, not hot, bath. Water that is too hot will cause the essential oils to dissipate. If you add milk to the water, it will prevent the oil from floating on top of the water and sticking to your skin. Soak as long as you are comfortable.

• • • •

# IBS (Irritable Bowel Syndrome)

There are many different ailments that are sometimes categorized as IBS. Allergies to foods, in particular, play a big part of being diagnosed with IBS, as does stress. Other ailments are often diagnosed as IBS, so keeping in close contact with your doctor is a must. Testing and diagnosis are the quickest way to treatment and to ensure that nothing more serious is at the root of the pain. IBS symptoms and pain can be reduced by applying various methods practiced around the world.

## AYURVEDA: *IBS Preventative*

In Ayurvedic medicine it is believed that all illness stems from the gut. One of the major contributors to illness in the digestive tract is stress. Managing stress is considered to be one of the best practices you can do for your body, and meditation is perhaps the greatest practice of all to manage stress.

To meditate, sit in a comfortable area outside on a porch, a quiet spot in your home, or in any area that you can relax and concentrate on yourself without any distractions such as phone or TV.

You may sit on a pillow if you cannot sit comfortably cross-legged. Cross your legs, keep your back straight, and rest your hands lightly on your knees.

Close your eyes and let your mind drift where it will. Do not concentrate on thinking about "nothing." Instead, concentrate on your breathing. When negative thoughts come, just brush them aside and go back to breathing.

Take deep, steady breaths in and out. Clean your lungs of old air and negativity and breathe in fresh air and positivity.

Repeat this cycle twice daily for five minutes. Add one minute each day until you can meditate for twenty minutes. This stress reliever will do wonders for your IBS, your spirit, your soul, and your life.

## HERB: *IBS Ointment*

This ointment provides the therapeutic properties to end the pain of IBS and bring a sense of comfort. Use sparingly, as a little goes a long way.

> ½ CUP PEPPERMINT LEAVES
>
> ½ CUP CHAMOMILE FLOWERS
>
> 1 TABLESPOON GRATED GINGER
>
> 1 CUP CARRIER OIL (SUCH AS JOJOBA, SESAME, GRAPESEED, OR YOUR PREFERENCE)
>
> 1–2 OUNCES BEESWAX
>
> 5 DROPS VITAMIN E OIL

Heat herbs, ginger, and carrier oil. Cook on very, very low heat in oven for one to three hours (225 to 300 degrees) or on extremely low heat on the stovetop. Strain. Compost or discard herbs. Add one to one and a half ounces of beeswax and the vitamin E oil to the herbal oil mixture, melt, and stir. Pour a drop of the ointment onto the countertop. Wait one minute and run a finger through the drop. If too thick, add more carrier oil; if too thin, add a little more beeswax. Pour mixture into a jar immediately, as it will harden quickly, and label. When cool, apply to affected area such as abdomen or lower back. Store in a cool, dark area for up to one year.

## ESSENTIAL OIL: *Digestive Pain Salve*

This treatment not only helps to end the pain of IBS, but it also contains calming oils that can help you to de-stress. Stress has been found to be a major contributor to IBS. Use this salve when you start to feel those first cramps or notice bloating.

> 3 TEASPOONS GRAPESEED OIL
>
> 1 TEASPOON BEESWAX
>
> 4 DROPS VITAMIN E OIL
>
> 3 DROPS GINGER OIL

3 DROPS CHAMOMILE OIL

3 DROPS PEPPERMINT OIL

In a small pan, heat the grapeseed oil and beeswax on the stovetop until just melted. Carefully remove the pan from heat and stir. Pour a drop of the melted oil and wax onto the counter and check the consistency after one minute. If it is too thin, add more beeswax; if it is too thick, add more grapeseed oil. Add the vitamin E and essential oils to the heated mixture. Whisk lightly; it will begin hardening immediately. Pour into containers. Once cool, apply to abdomen or lower back. Do not apply to mucus membranes, eyes, genitals, or open wounds. Label containers and store in a dark, dry area for up to one year.

### HOME REMEDY: *Dos and Don'ts for IBS*

Professionals work with a lot of IBS patients in helping them with pain management, managing stress, and ridding themselves of IBS. These are tips from the top professionals around the world. Try to incorporate some of these into your daily living practices.

- Take a probiotic at every meal. Probiotics work to rid us of harmful bacteria and replace it with good bacteria.

- Daily doses of fiber are paramount to maintaining a healthy digestive system for everyone, especially those with digestive tract issues.

- Getting the amount of sleep that you need for your body allows your energy to go toward helping your furnace burn your fuel. Don't short yourself on sleep.

- Eat smaller meals daily—no large, heavy meals. Do not eat fats, artificial sweeteners, cruciferous vegetables, candy, or unhealthy foods.

- Yoga has proven to be beneficial in helping end IBS. Yoga rids our body of deeply buried toxins, reduces stress, and gives our digestive tract a great workout.

- Any form of exercise, especially if done outdoors, improves our digestion, stress level, and mood.

• • • •
# JETLAG

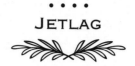

Jetlag is a very real condition. Feeling tired and worn out when on vacation is miserable. There are a lot of tips and recipes you can utilize to get you feeling energetic and happy again. Try some of these the next time you take off for that vacation of a lifetime!

## AYURVEDA: *Grounded While Flying*

Ayurveda believes that a vata imbalance is the main culprit in jet lag due to the body not being grounded while in the air. This recipe brings grounding while in the air and also after landing in that new continent.

### 1 TABLESPOON SESAME OIL

During your flight, use sesame oil on your throat, hands, and feet to give you the grounding you need while in the air. After landing, rub your entire body down with the oil. Let it soak in for ten minutes, then take a shower. You will reduce that feeling of disorientation that often accompanies people suffering from jet lag.

## HERB: *Tonic Tea*

This tea will give you the get-up-and-go needed to keep up when your body just wants to sleep. Getting into the new rhythm of day and night can be very disorienting. This tea will help you to wake up that sluggish mind and participate in your daily plans.

### 1 CUP WATER

### 1 PIECE OF GINSENG, DICED

### 1 TEASPOON PEPPERMINT

Bring water to a boil, then add herbs. Remove from heat, cover, and steep for six minutes. Strain and, if desired, add sweetener of choice.

## ESSENTIAL OIL: *Energy Bath*

Take this bath before you go out on the town and no one will know you just spent the last fourteen hours cramped up in a plane. These oils contain properties that work as a tonic to your body and soul.

**8 DROPS FRANKINCENSE OIL**

**8 DROPS BERGAMOT OIL**

**8 DROPS GRAPEFRUIT OIL**

**1 TABLESPOON CARRIER OIL (SUCH AS JOJOBA, SESAME, GRAPESEED, OR YOUR PREFERENCE)**

**1 TABLESPOON MILK (OPTIONAL)**

As you begin to fill the tub with water, pour the essential oils and carrier oil into the running water. Run a warm, not hot, bath. Water that is too hot will cause the essential oils to dissipate. If you add milk to the water, it will prevent the oil from floating on top of the water and sticking to your skin. Soak as long as you are comfortable to revive and renew your spirit!

## HOME REMEDY: *Jet Lag Diet*

During your flight and after you land, for twenty-four hours you should eat a diet high in protein during the day and high in carbohydrates at night. The protein during the day will give you energy; the carbohydrates at night will help you fall asleep easier. The time change is a huge culprit in causing jet lag, and your diet can get you back on track much quicker.

**Day:** Eat proteins such as fish, peanut butter, chicken, eggs, and cheese.

**Night:** Eat the carbs you dream of, such as pasta, potatoes, and corn. Remember to stay hydrated all day long.

• • • •

# JOINT PAIN

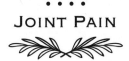

Overexertion, arthritis, illness, diet, age, weather, or any number of variables can cause joint pain. Easing that pain has been a quest since the beginning of time. These recipes, tips, and blends have been around for centuries, and the healing agents in the therapeutic properties bring quick pain relief.

## AYURVEDA: *Joint Massage Oil*

Ayurveda treatments for sore or swollen joints always include tea with turmeric in it. Turmeric is a powerful anti-inflammatory. Ayurvedic practitioners also deeply believe in massage. Try this massage treatment the next time your joints start to ache and pain you.

### 1–2 TABLESPOONS OLIVE OR SESAME OIL

Rub the oil into the affected areas. The oil should be slightly warm or at room temperature. The lubricant will ease your joints, and the massaging motion will help bring movement back to your joints. This practice should be performed morning and night.

## HERB: *Aspirin Tea*

Willow is the most powerful of analgesics. Try this tea when you wake up in the morning and when joint pain is at its worst. This will enable you to begin movement in the joints and regain flexibility.

### 1 CUP WATER

### 1 TEASPOON WHITE WILLOW BARK

### 1 TEASPOON MINT LEAVES

Bring water to a boil, then add herbs. Remove from heat, cover, and steep for ten to twelve minutes. Strain and, if desired, add sweetener of choice. Compost or discard herbs.

## ESSENTIAL OIL: *Oil Joint Rub*

These oils have anti-inflammatory, analgesic, antispasmodic, and antiarthritic compounds that ease pain, reduce swelling, and get you back on your feet again. Use this every day until that pain disappears.

### 10 DROPS PEPPERMINT OIL

### 10 DROPS EUCALYPTUS OIL

### 6 DROPS VITAMIN E OIL

### 2 OUNCES CARRIER OIL (SUCH AS JOJOBA, SESAME, GRAPESEED, OR YOUR PREFERENCE)

Mix the ingredients in a small glass container and apply lightly to the area desired, such as elbow, wrist, knees, and other painful joints. Keep essential oil mixture away from open wounds, mucus membranes, genitals, eyes, and sensitive areas. Repeat application as needed, usually two to three times daily. Store unused portion in a glass jar with a tight-fitting lid, label it, and keep it in a cool, dark area for up to six months.

## HOME REMEDY: *Pain-Relieving Bath*

This is the bath I take often when I have arthritis in my hips. It is soothing and enables me to get around well for the rest of the day or to sleep well at night. I like to add essential oils such as lavender, frankincense, juniper, or peppermint so that the healing properties can work alongside the salt to bring me relief.

¼ CUP EPSOM SALT

15 DROPS ESSENTIAL OILS OF CHOICE

1 TABLESPOON MILK (OPTIONAL)

As the bath water is running, add the Epsom salt to the water. Ensure that the water is not so hot that it will scald the skin. Once the tub is full, add the oils and milk, if desired. If you add milk to the water, it will prevent the oil from floating on top of the water and sticking to your skin. Relax completely in the tub for at least fifteen minutes to let the healing compounds perform their magic. Enjoy!

• • • •

# LARYNGITIS

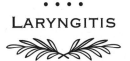

Laryngitis is disruptive and often the result of another illness but is not usually painful on its own. Occasionally, though, overuse of the voice box can result in laryngitis. These remedies will help you to get your voice back in tip-top shape in no time.

## AYURVEDA: *Onion Throat Syrup*

This easy-to-make remedy is often used in Ayurveda to bring relief to vocal cords. The onion is potent with antimicrobial properties and will help to bring your voice back to normal.

    1 CUP BOILING WATER

    1 ONION, CHOPPED

    3 TEASPOONS LEMON JUICE

    3 TABLESPOONS HONEY

Pour boiling water over the chopped onion and cover. Let the onions steep in the water for about twenty minutes. Strain the onion and discard. To the liquid, add the lemon and honey. Take teaspoons throughout the day as desired. Refrigerate any leftover in a covered container for up to twenty-four hours. It's best to warm slightly or take at room temperature.

## HERB: *Basil Throat Tea*

This herbal tea blend contains the properties needed to ward against illness, reduce swelling and inflammation, and relieve any pain. Drink up to three times daily.

    1 CUP WATER

    1 TEASPOON BASIL LEAVES

    1 TEASPOON THYME LEAVES

    LEMON JUICE (OPTIONAL)

Bring water to a boil, then add herbs. Remove from heat, cover, and steep for six to eight minutes. Strain and, if desired, add sweetener of choice. Compost or discard herbs. Adding lemon juice will also help to soothe and heal the throat area.

## ESSENTIAL OIL: *Throat-Relieving Air*

This blend contains oils that will help your throat muscles relax. The therapeutic properties of anti-inflammatory and antispasmodic agents will help to rid your body of any swelling or inflammation.

5 DROPS THYME OIL

5 DROPS CHAMOMILE OIL

5 DROPS SAGE OIL

WATER

Add oils and water to diffuser and run as desired.

### HOME REMEDY: *Laryngitis Tips*

These tips from various cultures are used daily because they work. Try to incorporate a few of these into your hourly or daily routines when suffering from laryngitis.

- Add lemon juice to all of your drinks or food. Lemons have a powerful component that will fight inflammation and infection as well as draw out toxins.

- The healthy, healing wonders of garlic cannot be emphasized enough. Add to your food or eat a piece raw.

- Gargle with a ¼ cup warm water that has 2 tablespoons salt in it. Spit out remainder, and do not swallow. Repeat three times daily.

- Add apple cider vinegar to drinks, salads, and vegetables. Take a teaspoon straight a couple times a day, if you can stand it.

- Honey is a great soother, not to mention all of the therapeutic properties it has that promote healing. Take honey several times a day in your drinks, food, or straight.

- Drink herbal teas throughout the day. Herbs carry healing properties that are chemical free and taste great.

- Breathe steam when possible. Soak in baths, take hot showers, or use a humidifier.

- Smoking aggravates the lining of the throat and the vocal cords. Smoking is a major contributor to laryngitis. Do not smoke.

- Speak softly, but don't whisper. Whispering uses the vocal cords more roughly than you may think. Try not to speak at all, but rest your voice.

• • • •

# LOW BLOOD PRESSURE (HYPOTENSION)

Having low blood pressure occasionally is common. But once it begins appearing often, it can lead to a medical emergency. It's best to be diagnosed by a professional to ascertain whether or not low blood pressure is caused by a more serious illness. Fainting, dizziness, nausea, and other symptoms may accompany hypotension. You should check with your doctor to ensure that none of the following recipes will interfere with your prescribed medications before embarking on a natural healing regimen for low blood pressure.

### AYURVEDA: *Pressure-Raising Chew*

This common Ayurvedic recipe raises the blood pressure and will have you feeling clear headed in the mornings. Many people suffer hypotension effects upon rising in the mornings. Having this blend ready will get you a good start to your day.

> 2 TABLESPOONS RAISINS
>
> 2 TABLESPOONS ALMONDS
>
> 1 CUP WATER

Soak the raisins and almonds in the water for six to eight hours or overnight. Slowly eat the raisins and the almonds—you can even drink the vitamin-enhanced water.

### HERB: *Hypotensive Tea*

Herbs have long been known to contain hypotensive properties. Drink this tea when you begin having that feeling of low blood pressure. Your pressure should rise, and you can experience the calming and healing effects of the tea. Ensure that this recipe does not conflict with any current medications.

> 1 CUP WATER
>
> ½ TEASPOON HOLY BASIL
>
> ½ TEASPOON LICORICE ROOT

**1 PINCH SALT**

**1 TEASPOON HONEY**

Bring water to a boil, then add herbs. Remove from heat, cover, and steep for six to eight minutes. Strain and add salt and honey. Compost or discard herbs.

### ESSENTIAL OIL: *Hypotensive Foot Drop*

Applying essential oils to the feet to increase or decrease blood pressure is a thousand-year-old practice. The oils are rapidly transmitted throughout the body and into the bloodstream, where hypotensive properties help to raise the blood pressure. Ensure that these oils do not interfere with your medications.

**2 DROPS ROSEMARY**

**2 DROPS SAGE**

**4 DROPS CARRIER OIL (SUCH AS JOJOBA, SESAME, GRAPESEED, OR YOUR PREFERENCE)**

Combine the oils into a spoon. With your fingertips, apply the oil to the soles of the feet. The oils will make your feet slippery, so wear socks or house shoes until the oils are absorbed into the skin.

### HOME REMEDY: *Hypotension Tips*

There are many common-sense ways to raise your blood pressure. Try to incorporate a few of these tips into your daily routine to keep your blood pressure at a good rate throughout the day.

- Eat salty foods and incorporate a pinch of salt into your drinks. Salt raises blood pressure.

- Change positions slowly, such as when you go from sitting to standing.

- Drink plenty of water every day. Getting dehydrated will certainly lower your blood pressure.

- Drink a cup of coffee when you feel your pressure starting to drop. Caffeine helps to raise blood pressure.

- Eat several small meals every day rather than two or three large meals. A large, heavy meal will raise your blood pressure, then it will bottom out, causing low blood pressure.

- Eat smaller portions of carbs, such as pasta, potatoes, and rice. These high-carb foods will cause your blood pressure to plummet.

• • • •
# MENOPAUSE
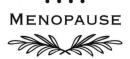

A decade-long change that affects every facet of a woman, menopause not only puts an end to the reproductive cycle, but its changes to our bodies, minds, and souls is profound. The menopause journey is one that may be faced with dread, prolonged by surprises, and end with a new chapter in our lives. The physical effects of menopause are uncomfortable, to say the least. These tips and recipes from around the world will help you to overcome many of the physical side effects of menopause.

## AYURVEDA: *Sheetali Pranayama (Cooling Breath)*

This is an ancient breathing treatment that instantly cools down the body. I have used this breathing technique many times for hot flashes, and it does work. Ayurvedic wisdom has many avenues to take in the quest for regulating menopause, but I love this one the most because you can do it anytime, anywhere, and it's free!

When having a hot flash, it's important to remove yourself from a hot area and into a cool area, such as moving out of the sun and into the shade. Find a cool area to sit in. If you're comfortable on the floor, cross your legs. Rest your hands on your knees and straighten your back. Form your tongue into a straw, or roll your tongue, then breathe in slowly through the circle formed by your tongue and breathe out slowly through your nose. Repeat this practice slowly twenty times, or until your body begins to cool off and the hot flash subsides. You will also find that you feel much calmer and more peaceful after completing this exercise.

## HERB: *Hormone Tincture*

This recipe contains herbs that are widely known for their abilities to reduce or eliminate many of the side effects of menopause such as bloating, mood swings, hot flashes, night sweats, and out-of-control eating.

**¾ PINT HIGH PROOF VODKA**

**2 TABLESPOONS CHASTE BERRIES**

**2 TABLESPOONS ST. JOHN'S WORT**

**2 TABLESPOONS RED CLOVER BLOSSOMS**

**2 TABLESPOONS SAGE LEAVES**

Place herbs in a pint jar until it's half full with dried herbs or two-thirds full with fresh herbs, and cover with a high proof vodka, about an inch from the top of the jar. Cover tightly and place in a cool, dark location. Shake vigorously every day for two weeks, then let it set without shaking for one month. Strain, bottle, and label, adding the date you decanted it (strained the herb). Use a half to one dropperful in tea, water, or other liquid. You can take it straight, though the taste is very strong. Tinctures made with alcohol will last up to three years if kept in a cool, dark place.

## ESSENTIAL OIL: *Hormone Balancing Spray*

This spray will calm you, cool you, and make things right with the world. Menopause often leads to horrific mood swings for no apparent reason. This spray will help you feel balanced and once again in control of your emotions.

**6 DROPS ANISE STAR OIL**

**6 DROPS YLANG-YLANG OIL**

**6 DROPS ANGELICA OIL**

**1 TEASPOON WITCH HAZEL**

**2 OUNCES WATER**

Add all ingredients to a dark-colored spray bottle to prevent sunlight from damaging contents. Shake bottle and spray onto area desired, such as body, hair, home, car, or office. Do not spray into open wounds, genitals, eyes, or mucus membranes. Store in a cool, dark area for up to three months. Shake well before each use to combine the ingredients.

## HOME REMEDY: *Natural Menopause Tips*

These hints and menopause life-savers have been passed down for generations all over the world. See which ones you would like to incorporate into your daily practice.

- Drink all the herbal tea you want. You can find teas to balance hormones, cool you off, calm you, and for all of the millions of emotions you will have during menopause.

- Vitamins A, B, D, and E all play a vital role in our continuing effort to maintain good health during menopause. A good multivitamin is very beneficial.

- Yoga works on the body, spirit, and mind, all of which need boosting during menopause. You can get really great results with the poses of downward facing dog, forward bend, and boat pose.

- Eliminate stress from your daily grind as often as possible.

- This is possibly one of the greatest tips about menopause: gaining weight before and after menopause is inevitable, but you can curb it by getting your daily amount of stress-reducing, feel-good exercise.

- Prayer and meditation are invaluable to a woman during this time of her life. I discovered meditation as I was going through menopause, and I am convinced it kept me from doing anything drastic!

- Drink ice water as much as you can to cool off your body.

- People swear by the compounds in soy for menopause. Soy is supposedly one of the best hormone balancers in existence.

- Your sleep may be disrupted up to a hundred times a night by hot flashes or night sweats. Try going to bed a little earlier and making up for all that sleep you will lose during the night.

• • • •

## Menstrual Cramps

Every woman experiences menstrual cramps during some point in their lives. Some of them are small and uncomfortable; sometimes they are debilitating. Learning to manage the pain associated with cramps is something we go through from a very early age. Using these techniques from around the world can give you different options to try during that monthly grind.

### AYURVEDA: *Cramp Tea and a Chaser*

This Ayurvedic recipe helps to reduce inflammation and spasms of the abdomen. It is quite soothing.

- 1 CUP WATER
- 1 TEASPOON GROUND GINGER
- 1 DASH CINNAMON
- 1 TEASPOON HONEY
- ½ TEASPOON FLAXSEED

Bring water to a boil, then add herbs. Remove from heat, cover, and steep for six to eight minutes. Strain and add honey. Compost or discard herbs. After drinking the tea, follow up by chewing on the flaxseed and swallowing. All of the components of this tea and chaser work together to bring you quick relief.

### HERB: *Herbal Cramp Balm*

This balm has always been a favorite of the women in my family. It's easy to have on hand, soothing, and it works! Keep a jar made up and handy so that the next time you get hit with those "double-me-over" cramps, relief will be at hand.

1 CUP OLIVE OR SESAME OIL

1 TABLESPOON GRATED GINGER

½ CUP BASIL LEAVES

1 TEASPOON FENNEL SEEDS

1 CINNAMON STICK

¼ TEASPOON VITAMIN E OIL

1 OUNCE BEESWAX

Put oil in a glass or stainless-steel pan and heat on very, very low. Add ginger, basil, fennel seeds, and the cinnamon to the oil. Stir, lower heat to warm, and let simmer for one hour. Strain through cheesecloth into jar. Add vitamin E oil and beeswax and stir until wax is dissolved. Pour into desired container. Label and date. Cool completely before using. Rub a small amount onto abdominal area for cramps. Do not get into eyes, genitals, mucus membranes, or sensitive areas. Store in a cool, dark area in a covered container for up to six months.

### ESSENTIAL OIL: *Soothing Cramp Bath Salts*

Make these bath salts ahead of time so they will be ready when you need them. These essential oils have antispasmodic, calming, anti-inflammatory properties to help ease those abdominal muscles and end your cramping. These jars make attractive, inexpensive, and healing gifts!

10 DROPS CLARY SAGE OIL

10 DROPS MARJORAM OIL

5 DROPS LAVENDER OIL

5 DROPS VITAMIN E OIL

2 TABLESPOONS CARRIER OIL (SUCH AS JOJOBA, SESAME, GRAPESEED, OR YOUR PREFERENCE)

3 CUPS SALTS (PINK HIMALAYAN, SEA, EPSOM, OR YOUR PREFERENCE)

1 TABLESPOON MILK (OPTIONAL)

Add the oils to the salt. Stir until well blended. Cover tightly. Leave mixture in a dark area for twenty-four hours, then stir mixture again. Run the bathwater, but not so hot as to ruin the oils. Add a half cup of the bath salt mixture to bathwater. If you add milk to the water, it will prevent the oil from floating on top of the water and sticking to your skin. Store unused portion in a glass jar with a tight-fitting lid, label it, and keep it in a cool, dark area for up to three months.

HOME REMEDY: *Cramp-Reducing Tips*

There are hundreds of cramp remedies that have been passed down from mother to daughter for thousands of years. Here is a list of the most-used remedies and how to avoid or end cramps:

- Place a heating pad on your abdomen for up to fifteen minutes at a time. Heat causes the muscles to relax.

- There are so many vitamins and minerals that can help to ease your cramps, so taking a multivitamin can get them all in. The iron helps replace the iron that is lost through blood flow every month.

- Herbs are loaded with anti-inflammatory and antispasmodic ingredients, as well as natural analgesics and uterine properties.

- Having an orgasm actually can end or temporarily relieve cramps.

- Have olive oil or good fats, such as in avocado, but try to stay away from fats as much as you can during menstruation. Bacon and cheeseburgers are tasty, but the animal fats cause inflammation, which leads to more cramping.

- Try to avoid using harsh chemicals for cleaning and other activities. Chemicals cause inflammation in the body and induce cramping.

- Try to get a good night's sleep and nap during the day if you can.

- Science shows us that exercise reduces the inflammation in our bodies. You may not be able to exercise during menstruation, but it works well if you keep your body toned and fit the rest of the month.

- Try doing some slow yoga stretches. Science has proven that yoga can help to reduce inflammation and spasms and end cramping.

· · · ·
# MIGRAINE

I have several family members who suffer from migraine headaches. Science does not know why some people get them and some people don't. The migraine headache has been around forever—and so have cures and pain relievers associated with them. Here I have gathered up several recipes from around the world; you can mix them up and try the different ingredients until you find the right combination that works for you.

## AYURVEDA: *Migraine Poultice*

This recipe is over five thousand years old and is still used today in India and other parts of the world. The properties in these ancient recipes are absorbed by the skin and delivered straight to those narrowed blood vessels. Reduce the pain of your next migraine by applying ingredients available right in your own kitchen!

### 1 HANDFUL OF LEMON SLICES, CABBAGE LEAVES, OR A SLICED POTATO

Wrap the ingredient you choose in a thin layer of damp gauze or linen. Apply to forehead and leave on for one hour. Discard after usage. You may reapply as often as you wish.

## HERB: *Migraine Herbal Tea*

These herbs all contain anti-inflammatory, antispasmodic, cephalic, and some analgesic properties for pain management. Choose two of the herbs and use one teaspoon of each to make the blend that works best for you.

### 1 CUP WATER

### 2 HERBS: FEVERFEW, WHITE WILLOW, VALERIAN ROOT, MULLEIN, YARROW, CHICKWEED, CHAMOMILE, OR GINGER

Bring water to a boil, then add herbs. Remove from heat, cover, and steep for six to eight minutes. Strain and, if desired, add sweetener of choice and lemon. Compost or discard herbs.

## ESSENTIAL OIL: *Migraine Essential Oil Diffuser*

This diffuser recipe will do more than diffuse the air. The anti-inflammatory and antispasmodic properties will also diffuse that migraine and make it go away. Use a combination of two or three of the following essential oils to make a blend that works on your personal migraine.

> 6–10 DROPS TOTAL OF ANY COMBINATION OF THE
> FOLLOWING OILS: ANGELICA, BASIL, FRANKINCENSE,
> HONEYSUCKLE, LAVENDER, LINDEN BLOSSOM,
> MARJORAM, PEPPERMINT, ROSEMARY, SPIKENARD,
> OR VALERIAN
>
> WATER

Add oils and water to diffuser and run as desired.

## HOME REMEDY: *Migraine Remedies*

Everybody's mom has a migraine cure that they are willing to share. I have collected a ton of these recipes, hints, and tips. Incorporating a few of these tips into your lifestyle could very well put an end to your migraines forever.

- Flaxseed is high in the vitamins that are proven to reduce or end migraines. Chew on a spoonful of flaxseed or add to salads and vegetables.

- Stay hydrated. Drink plenty of water and all sorts of herbal teas. The caffeine in green tea has been proven to help open narrowed blood vessels and reduce migraine pain.

- Do whatever you need to do to get rid of the stress in your life: pray, meditate, walk in nature, go fishing...

- Ensuring you get eight hours of sleep a night has been shown to dramatically reduce the incidence of migraines for many people.

- Yoga has been proven to reduce migraines altogether. Try some slow, easy poses at first and work your way up to a full-blown regimen.

- Take a multivitamin every day. Vitamins help keep the blood flowing and will help you stay healthy.

- No nitrates: no hot dogs, lunch meat, or sausages.

- Give yourself a massage—or, better yet, get someone else to give you one. Use sesame oil or a light oil mixed with essential oils to get those therapeutic properties incorporated into your blood.

- Complete the elimination diet. Eliminate a food such as dairy, gluten, or chocolate (or sweets of any kind) for two weeks, then see whether your migraines are triggered once you incorporate a certain food group back into your diet.

• • • •

# MOTION SICKNESS

Motion sickness can ruin even the most pleasant of trips. Nausea, vomiting, headaches, sinus pain, and dizziness can be signs that you are suffering from motion sickness. Recipes, tips, and hints from different cultures can help you overcome this annoying condition. Try a couple of these each time you have to sail, fly, or drive to put an end to that discomfort once and for all.

## AYURVEDA: *Motion Sickness Drink*

In India this is a common treatment for motion sickness. It is simple, and the ingredients are already in your refrigerator. Limes are known for their nausea-reducing qualities.

**1 TABLESPOON LIME JUICE**

**¼ CUP WATER**

Pour the lime juice into a container of water, cover tightly, and shake well. Let sit for one hour at room temperature. Shake well again, and drink slowly throughout your trip.

## HERB: *Motion Tea*

This is probably the oldest and most-used motion sickness diversion tactic. Ginger is used worldwide to end nausea and dizziness. The added benefit of the fennel seeds works well in conjunction with the ginger to double the healing properties.

1 CUP WATER

½-INCH GINGER ROOT, MINCED

½ TEASPOON FENNEL SEEDS

Bring water to a boil, then add herbs. Remove from heat, cover, and steep for ten to twelve minutes. Strain and, if desired, add sweetener of choice. Compost or discard herbs.

## ESSENTIAL OIL: *Motion Inhale*

Some people swear by peppermint essential oil inhalation as a cure for motion sickness (and other types of nausea as well). It's easy to keep a small vial of peppermint handy in your car or purse for when that uneasy feeling begins to strike.

2 DROPS PEPPERMINT OIL

Apply oil to palm of hand, oil inhaler, or tissue, bring it close to your nostrils, and inhale the aroma deeply. This process sends the properties straight to your brain, and the effects are immediate.

## HOME REMEDY: *Motion Sickness Prevention*

These tips and hints are used in various cultures to prevent motion sickness. Try a few of these the next time you take a trip and see what works for you.

- Eating a clove of garlic quells nausea in many people, and you just might be one of them. Your fellow passengers may take offense, though.

- Focus on a focal point, lift your head, and stare straight ahead. Try to move your head as little as possible.

- Sit in the front seat or on the top deck when possible.

- Use a fan or crack a window to blow the cool air in your face. This often helps to calm the stomach.

- Drink ginger ale, herbal teas, green tea, and water. Stay hydrated.

- Incorporate crackers, apple juice, lemons, marjoram, and peppermint into your diet before your trip.

- Breathe in and out slowly and with deep breaths. Deep breathing will relax all your muscles and help you to avoid stomach spasms.

- Listen to music or concentrate on something besides feeling sick.

. . . .

# MUSCLES/LIGAMENTS/TENDON PAIN

Arthritis, overexertion, weather, or bumps and bruises are a few of the reasons that someone might suffer with pain in their muscles, ligaments, and tendons. After ascertaining that a serious injury has not caused the pain, you can indulge in one of these soothing, healing treatments from cultures around the world. If the pain is intense or lingers, then it's time to seek medical attention.

### AYURVEDA: *Pain Tea*

In Ayurvedic medicine adding turmeric to your food and drinks is the number one way of eliminating inflammation. Try this tea to ease the pain and discomfort of your aching muscles. The properties at work here are both anti-inflammatory and antispasmodic.

 1 CUP WATER

 ½ TEASPOON GROUND VALERIAN ROOT

 ½ TEASPOON CHAMOMILE FLOWERS

 ½ TEASPOON TURMERIC

Bring water to a boil, then add the valerian and chamomile. Remove from heat, cover, and steep for six to eight minutes. Strain and, if desired, add sweetener of choice. Add turmeric and stir. Compost or discard herbs.

## HERB: *Pain Balm*

These herbs contain anti-inflammatory and anti-spasmodic therapeutic properties and help to ease pain and discomfort, as well as any inflammation.

1 CUP OLIVE OR SESAME OIL

1 TABLESPOON VALERIAN ROOT, GROUND

½ CUP SAGE LEAVES

½ CUP DEVIL'S CLAW

1 OUNCE BEESWAX

5 DROPS VITAMIN E OIL

Put olive or sesame oil in a glass or stainless-steel pan over very, very low heat. Add crushed and ground herbs and stir. Let simmer for one hour. Strain through cheesecloth into jar. Add beeswax and vitamin E oil and stir until wax is dissolved. Pour into desired container. Label and date. Cool completely before using. To use, apply a thin layer to the painful area and rub it in. You may cover the area with a light gauze if clothing or furniture need protecting. Do not apply to mucus membranes, genitals, eyes, or sensitive areas. Store in a covered container for up to six months in a cool, dry area.

## ESSENTIAL OIL: *Pain Rub*

These oils work well with their analgesic and pain-reducing therapeutic properties. You must complete a patch test before using these essential oils as wintergreen and birch oils in particular are very powerful. Conduct the patch test by mixing a drop of the essential oil with eight drops of carrier oil. Apply to your skin and leave on for twelve hours. Check at the end of twelve hours to ensure that your skin is not red, itching, blistered, or in any way harmed by the essential oil. If you do notice any skin irritation, then do not use that particular oil in any way.

10 DROPS WINTERGREEN OIL

8 DROPS BIRCH OIL

8 DROPS PEPPERMINT OIL

6 DROPS VITAMIN E OIL

1 OUNCE CARRIER OIL (SUCH AS JOJOBA, SESAME, GRAPESEED, OR YOUR PREFERENCE)

Mix the ingredients in a small glass container and apply lightly to the area desired, such as muscles, ligaments, and tendons. Keep essential oil mixture away from open wounds, mucus membranes, genitals, eyes, and sensitive areas. Repeat application as needed, usually two to three times daily. Store unused portion in a glass jar with a tight-fitting lid, label it, and keep it in a cool, dark area for up to six months.

### HOME REMEDY: *Pain Bath*

This is an all-around favorite remedy for achy and painful muscles, ligaments, and tendons. This simple recipe works well due to the magnesium content of the Epsom salt that is directly responsible for easing pain in the joints and muscles. The hot water in the bath is a soothing accompaniment to double your relief.

Add one cup Epsom salt to the running water. Ensure that the water is not so hot that it will cause your skin to burn or dry out. You may soak in the water as long as you are comfortable—twenty minutes is the recommended time.

· · · ·

# NAUSEA

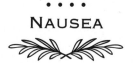

There aren't many worse feelings than nausea, which is often accompanied by a host of unwanted effects: dizziness, cramping, vomiting, headaches—the list is endless. There are countless reasons why a person might suffer from nausea. You can either let it run its course or try some of these well-known remedies. If nausea continues and leads to dehydration, a trip to the ER may be in order to determine the cause and to treat dehydration.

### AYURVEDA: *Nausea Rice Water*

Ayurvedic practitioners are firm believers in rice water for nausea. Jasmine or basmati rice are great varieties to use for this recipe. Rice water works wonders in soothing the stomach and aids in healing the digestive tract.

1 CUP RICE

WATER

PINCH OF SALT

Prepare the rice and salt according to package directions, except add an extra one and a half cups of water. This will leave the rice with an excess of water once it has completed cooking. Strain the rice and pour the rice water into a glass. Once the water has cooled, slowly sip it. Your stomach will settle quickly. Keep the rice in the refrigerator for up to three days and eat it once you are feeling better.

## HERB: *Natural Ginger Syrup*

Ginger ale has been the go-to drink for years in combatting nausea. Make your own version of ginger ale with a few simple items. Ginger has antiemetic, antispasmodic, and anti-inflammatory properties to soothe a stomach.

2–2½ CUPS GINGER ROOT

4 CUPS WATER

¾ CUP SUGAR

1 TABLESPOON LIME JUICE

CLUB SODA

Mince the ginger and add to a pan. Add water and bring to a boil. Reduce heat and simmer lightly for fifteen minutes. Add the sugar and continue to simmer for twenty minutes. Remove from heat and add the lime juice. Cool slightly and strain. Discard the herb. When ready to drink, add one cup of club soda to one-fourth cup ginger syrup. Refrigerate up to seven days.

## ESSENTIAL OIL: *Tummy Soother*

These essential oils contain antiemetic properties to ease nausea, cramping, and spasms. Try this rub on your tummy the next time you are trying to keep it all down.

**10 DROPS PEPPERMINT OIL**

**10 DROPS FENNEL OIL**

**2 OUNCES CARRIER OIL (SUCH AS JOJOBA, SESAME, GRAPESEED, OR YOUR PREFERENCE)**

**4 DROPS VITAMIN E OIL**

Mix the ingredients in a small glass container and apply lightly to the area desired, such as abdomen and lower back. Keep essential oil mixture away from open wounds, mucus membranes, genitals, eyes, and sensitive areas. Repeat application as needed, usually two to three times daily. Store unused portion in a glass jar with a tight-fitting lid, label it, and keep it in a cool, dark area for up to six months.

**HOME REMEDY:** *Queasy Lemon Calmer*

Lemon has long been known for its antiemetic, anti-inflammatory, and anti-spasmodic properties. Omit the salt if you suffer from high blood pressure.

**1 TABLESPOON FRESH LEMON JUICE**

**¼ TEASPOON SALT**

**8 OUNCES WATER**

Combine the ingredients together in a glass. Sip slowly until nausea passes. You may keep remainder in the refrigerator for up to twenty-four hours.

• • • •

# NECK PAIN

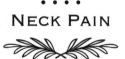

The neck holds up the head, and that is never more evident than when the neck is in pain. The head begins to feel as if it weighs a thousand pounds. Relieve neck pain quickly with these recipes and blends. If neck pain persists, ensure through your medical advisor that it is not the result of a more serious condition than just sore muscles.

## AYURVEDA: *Neck Easing*

In Ayurveda it is believed that neck pain is a stress signal to the body. Try incorporating gentle asanas (yoga poses) into your routine such as corpse pose. Eat a soothing diet and use the following anti-inflammatory massage oil on the neck daily.

½ TEASPOON GINGER, FINELY DICED

½ TEASPOON VALERIAN ROOT, FINELY DICED

1 OUNCE SESAME OIL

½ TEASPOON TURMERIC POWDER

In a small pan, mix the ginger and valerian together with the oil. Heat on very low for twenty minutes. Strain the mixture. Add the turmeric powder, stir to blend, and cool. Using fingertips, rub onto neck in a gentle circular motion. Do not apply mixture to mucus membranes, eyes, genitals, mouth, wounds, or sensitive areas. Wipe off excess with a towel. Store unused portion in a glass jar with a tight-fitting lid, label it, and keep it in a cool, dark area for up to three months.

## HERB: *Herbal Pain Ointment*

This blend has been used forever to reduce inflammation and ease the pain of a stiff and achy neck. The anti-inflammatory properties reduce swelling and have antispasmodic agents to end spasms.

1 OUNCE LAVENDER FLOWERS

1 OUNCE ST. JOHN'S WORT

1 CUP OLIVE OIL

½ TEASPOON VITAMIN E OIL

1 OUNCE BEESWAX

Mix the herbs and olive oil and cook on very, very low heat in the oven for one to three hours or on extremely low heat on the stovetop. Strain, add vitamin E oil and beeswax, and stir well until wax has melted. Pour mixture into a jar, cool, and apply as a rub to neck and shoulders. You may wish to cover with a bandage, linen, or light cloth as the ointment will stain clothing and furniture. Store unused portion in a glass jar with a tight-fitting lid, label it, and keep it in a cool, dark area for up to one year.

## ESSENTIAL OIL: *Stiff Neck Ease*

A stiff neck can be a real pain! Ease into the day by rubbing this blend on your neck. The antispasmodic, anti-inflammatory, and analgesic properties are absorbed by the skin into the areas of the neck that need the most magic.

- 5 DROPS WINTERGREEN OIL

- 5 DROPS FRANKINCENSE OIL

- 3 DROPS THYME OIL

- 3 DROPS PEPPERMINT OIL

- 1 OUNCE CARRIER OIL (SUCH AS JOJOBA, SESAME, GRAPESEED, OR YOUR PREFERENCE)

- 4 DROPS VITAMIN E OIL

Mix the ingredients in a small glass container and apply lightly to the area desired, such as the neck or throat area. Keep essential oil mixture away from open wounds, mucus membranes, genitals, eyes, and sensitive areas. Repeat application as needed, usually two to three times daily. Store unused portion in a glass jar with a tight-fitting lid, label it, and keep it in a cool, dark area for up to six months.

## HOME REMEDY: *Cold/Hot Pain Remedy*

This old-fashioned home remedy does wonders for neck pain and other pain from strain or stress. You will need a cloth to hold crushed ice and a heating pad. Try this for about fifteen minutes out of every hour and you will be surprised at how well it works in most cases.

While relaxing comfortably, apply a cloth or bag filled with ice to the neck area. Leave ice on for eight minutes or for however long it is comfortable. Do not leave on too long or the ice will burn your skin. Once you remove the ice, then apply a heating pad to your neck or get in the shower and let the hot water (not too hot!) stream onto your neck. Heat the neck for eight minutes while in a comfortable position. Repeat the process every hour until neck pain dissipates.

· · · ·

# NERVE PAIN (NEURALGIA)

Nerve pain can sometimes be debilitating and excruciatingly painful. There are numerous reasons why a person would suffer nerve pain. Neuralgia commonly affects people over the age of fifty and more women than men. It is said to be so painful that people have trouble talking. Always consult a physician to rule out more serious diseases. Neuralgia can often be treated with medications that can assist greatly in reducing or even eliminating pain. Essential oils, herbs, Ayurveda, and home remedies have been used for centuries to reduce nerve pain.

## AYURVEDA: *Neuralgia Air*

In India the smoke from thyme, sage, and cloves often fills the air to dispel nerve pain. When you have the whole herb, you could smudge it with sage to enhance the air with the healing components.

**3 THYME STEMS**

**1 SAGE SMUDGE STICK**

Wrap the thyme stems around the sage smudge stick. Light the end, carefully holding over a plate so that the embers won't fall on the carpet or floor. Carefully fan the smoke away from your body while walking from room to room. Think positive and healthy thoughts and wishes as you pray while traveling into each room. Don't put the smudge stick down anywhere except in a glass or metal dish.

## HERB: *Nerve Tea*

This herbal concoction has been used for centuries in the treatment of nerve pain. The properties in the herbs soothe and relax the nerves and also give you an overall feeling of well-being. It has been said that drinking this tea daily will help to heal nerve pain altogether.

1 CUP WATER

½ TEASPOON ST. JOHN'S WORT

½ TEASPOON PEPPERMINT LEAVES

Bring water to a boil, then add herbs. Remove from heat, cover, and steep for six to eight minutes. Strain and, if desired, add sweetener of choice. Compost or discard herbs.

## ESSENTIAL OIL: *Neuralgia Massage*

These essential oils are said to be very comforting. If used repeatedly, they can often put an end to nerve pain altogether. The anti-inflammatory and antispasmodic properties work together to stop nerve pain.

10 DROPS EUCALYPTUS OIL

10 DROPS CHAMOMILE OIL

5 DROPS HELICHRYSUM OIL

5 DROPS CLOVE OIL

1 OUNCE CARRIER OIL (SUCH AS JOJOBA, SESAME, GRAPESEED, OR YOUR PREFERENCE)

4 DROPS VITAMIN E OIL

Mix ingredients in a glass container and lightly massage the area desired, such as the temples, neck, chest, back, soles of feet, or painful nerve areas. Keep essential oil mixture away from open wounds, mucus membranes, genitals, eyes, and sensitive areas. Repeat application as needed. Store unused portion in a glass jar with a tight-fitting lid, label it, and keep it in a cool, dark area for up to three months.

## HOME REMEDY: *Neuralgia Juice Remedy*

Sometimes home remedies are the easiest *and* the yummiest! Try this juice, which helps to quell nerve pain with its anti-inflammatory and antispasmodic properties. Drink this blend at least once daily until pain is gone.

½ APPLE, CORED

1 CARROT

1 CELERY STALK

½ CUP LIQUID (JUICE, TEA, OR WATER)

Combine ingredients together in a blender. Blend until it is of a smooth drinking consistency. Drink cold or at room temperature.

· · · ·

# NOSEBLEED

Minor nosebleeds happen in young children for no apparent reason. As long as the bleeding stops within a few minutes, home remedies and other methods can be of use. If bleeding continues or is extremely heavy, medical assistance should be sought. Adults can get nosebleeds, too, and the reasons are limitless. Sinus infections, bumps, headaches, and other conditions can cause even the healthiest of us to have a nosebleed. These remedies have been used throughout time to staunch the flow.

### AYURVEDA: *Ice Treatment*

While this recipe seems very simple, it is also quite effective at stopping the flow of blood. Ice slows down the flow of blood and will end a nosebleed pretty quickly.

Place crushed ice inside a cloth and apply to the bridge of your nose. Sit up straight and tilt your head back, resting it on top of a chair or the couch. The blood will cool rapidly, and the flow will ebb.

## HERB: *Astringent Wash*

The astringent and hemostatic properties in these herbs work to help narrow the blood vessels and stop the flow of blood from the nose.

½ TEASPOON MINT LEAVES

½ TEASPOON YARROW

½ TEASPOON AGRIMONY

1 CUP BOILING WATER

Place the herbs into the boiling water. Remove from heat, cover, and steep for ten minutes. Strain and discard herbs. Once mixture is cool enough, use a cotton swab or cloth and dip it into the liquid. Apply wet cloth to outer nose and wash gently while tilting head back. Discard any remainder after twenty-four hours.

## ESSENTIAL OIL: *Lemon Inhale*

No one seems to know why the smell of lemons can stop a nosebleed, but it often does. This is easy, quick, and can be done in a moment's notice.

1–2 DROPS LEMON ESSENTIAL OIL

Apply oil to palm of hand, oil inhaler, or tissue, bring close to your nostrils, and inhale the aroma deeply. This process sends the properties straight to your brain, and the effects are immediate. You can repeat this procedure as needed.

## HOME REMEDY: *Cotton Ball for Nosebleeds*

This old home remedy works well to stop blood flow. These ingredients are usually already in your cupboard and very cheap to purchase. It's quick, easy, and effective.

½ TEASPOON VINEGAR OR WITCH HAZEL

1 COTTON BALL

Place the liquid on the cotton ball. Place the cotton ball gently into the outer nostril and let sit for ten minutes. Do not apply to open wounds, genitals, or other sensitive areas. Repeat as needed. Discard cotton ball once completed.

. . . .

# OCD (Obsessive Compulsive Disorder)

When a person has the same thoughts of worry over and over, this is a type of obsessive compulsive disorder, or OCD. There are many types of OCD, and these thought patterns are very hard to break. Locking and unlocking doors repeatedly, washing the hands repeatedly, or counting and repeating words are all forms of OCD. New medications offer hope and wellness to many who have suffered from chronic OCD. Therapy has also proved to be very useful in treating OCD patients. Essential oils, herbs, Ayurveda, and home remedies can be used to bring calmness to a situation where someone suffering from OCD could have troubling or life-altering situations.

### AYURVEDA: *Ashwagandha Milk*

Ashwagandha is used in Ayurvedic medicine to treat all types of brain disorders, stress disorders, ADHD, OCD, and any disorder where it is believed that better circulation of the blood to the brain will help to quell problems. This little drink, taken at bedtime, will help you to relax, be calm, and sleep soundly. The flavor is superb, and the benefits are remarkable.

1 TEASPOON ASHWAGANDHA POWDER

½ TEASPOON HONEY

1 CUP MILK

Mix ingredients together and drink warm or cold.

### HERB: *OCD Tea*

When used in combination, St. John's wort and ginkgo biloba can drastically reduce stress, nervousness, vata, anxiety, and OCD actions. The wonderful properties make this the perfect tea to drink every day when dealing with any of those hyper mental activities.

1 CUP WATER

½ TEASPOON GINKGO BILOBA LEAVES

½ TEASPOON ST. JOHN'S WORT LEAVES OR BUDS

Bring water to a boil, then add herbs. Remove from heat, cover, and steep for six to eight minutes. Strain and, if desired, add sweetener of choice and lemon. Compost or discard herbs.

## ESSENTIAL OIL: *OCD Rub*

This recipe has essential oils that calm the mind and the body. A relaxed state is very important when trying to overcome OCD. When the repetitive habits are out of control, rub on this mixture and you will begin to calm down enough to concentrate on other tasks besides that repetitive habit.

**10 DROPS CYPRESS OIL**

**8 DROPS FRANKINCENSE OIL**

**8 DROPS YLANG-YLANG OIL**

**5 DROPS VITAMIN E OIL**

**2 OUNCES CARRIER OIL (SUCH AS JOJOBA, SESAME, GRAPESEED, OR YOUR PREFERENCE)**

Mix the ingredients in a small glass container and apply lightly to the area desired, such as pressure points, neck, soles of feet, temples, and chest. Keep essential oil mixture away from open wounds, mucus membranes, genitals, eyes, and sensitive areas. Repeat application as needed, usually two to three times daily. Store unused portion in a glass jar with a tight-fitting lid, label it, and keep it in a cool, dark area for up to six months.

## HOME REMEDY: *OCD Home Remedies*

Thousands of people have incorporated a few of these tips into their daily lives and have had success with completely eliminating all of their OCD tendencies. It may just work for you, too. Try including a couple of tips a day for a few weeks and then see what your outcome is.

- No smoking or tobacco of any kind.
- No alcohol.
- Take hot baths at night instead of a shower.
- Get at least seven or eight hours of sleep a night.

- Do whatever kind of exercise you want, but don't be sedentary. Take up yoga, ride a bike, swim.

- Eat three well-balanced, healthy meals a day. Don't skip meals. Try to stay away from sugar, caffeine, or any food that anyone in your family is allergic to.

- Go outdoors—winter or summer, it doesn't matter. Sunshine, vitamin D, fresh air, and nature are all imperative to having a healthy mind.

- Pray, chant, and do whatever stress-reducing, faith-fulfilling, joy-inducing activity you can to help you in your journey to good mental health.

• • • •

# PANIC ATTACKS

Panic attacks are frightening and can mimic hysteria, heart attacks, and pain. The attack can manifest itself in many different ways, for many different reasons. Getting calm is the number one goal during the attack. Natural remedies from around the planet can help with this as well as for preventing further attacks.

## AYURVEDA: *Panic to Peace Massage*

In Ayurveda these herbs are well known for their ability to calm, reduce anxiety, increase longevity, increase brain power, and induce feelings of well-being. Sesame oil is used for its warming and grounding benefits. Ayurvedic medicine teaches us that when you have anxiety or panic attacks, you should get as warm and comfortable as you can.

1 TEASPOON ASHWAGANDHA POWDER

1 TEASPOON BRAHMI POWDER

4 OUNCES SESAME OIL

6 DROPS VITAMIN E OIL

Place the ashwagandha and brahmi powders in a small saucepan along with the sesame oil. Cook over very low heat for twenty minutes, until the herbs are blended into the oil. Remove from heat and add the vitamin E oil. Cool until room temperature. Apply to soles of feet, temples, or neck area. Mixture can be used as a massage oil over the entire body. Store unused portion in a glass jar with a tight-fitting lid, label it, and keep it in a cool, dark area for up to three months.

### HERB: *Fortifying Balm*

The more you use this balm daily, the less your panic attacks will sneak up on you. These herbs have calming, relaxing, and fortifying properties to rid you of anxiety and get you prepared to face the world.

> 1 OUNCE CARRIER OIL (SUCH AS JOJOBA, SESAME, GRAPESEED, OR YOUR PREFERENCE)
>
> ½ OUNCE PASSION FLOWER PETALS
>
> ½ OUNCE LEMON BALM LEAVES
>
> 6 DROPS VITAMIN E OIL
>
> 1 OUNCE BEESWAX

Put carrier oil in a glass or stainless-steel pan and heat on very low. Add crushed herbs and stir. Simmer slowly over low heat for one hour. Strain through cheesecloth into jar. Discard herbs. Add beeswax and stir until wax is dissolved. Add vitamin E oil. Pour into desired container. Label and date. Cool completely before using. Rub on temples, back of neck, chest, soles of feet, or other areas. Do not apply to eyes, ears, mucus membranes, open wounds, or sensitive areas. Store in covered container in a cool, dark area, for up to six months.

### ESSENTIAL OIL: *Breathe Deep Bath*

Studies have shown that increased usage of these essential oils significantly reduces panic attacks. Relax in this sweet-smelling bath and let your anxiety dissipate.

> 6 DROPS LEMON BALM (MELISSA) OIL
>
> 6 DROPS CHAMOMILE OIL

6 DROPS LAVENDER OIL

1 TABLESPOON CARRIER OIL (SUCH AS JOJOBA, SESAME, GRAPESEED, OR YOUR PREFERENCE)

1 TABLESPOON MILK (OPTIONAL)

As you begin to fill the tub with water, pour the essential oils and carrier oil into the running water. Run a warm, not hot, bath. Water that is too hot will cause the essential oils to dissipate. If you add milk to the water, it will prevent the oil from floating on top of the water and sticking to your skin. Soak in the water as long as you are comfortable.

### HOME REMEDY: *Panic-Reducing Tips*

Most of these tips have been used since the Middle Ages to reduce panic attacks and anxiety. The reason they have been practiced for so long is because they work! Try incorporating a few of these tips into your life daily and watch your incidences of attacks decrease or vanish altogether.

- There is nothing else like the calming, powerful feeling of taking a walk in the woods, sitting on the green earth, or watching ducks on a pond. Get outside daily, no matter the weather, and marvel at the wonder of nature.

- Take your daily vitamins. B6 and niacin are great anxiety inhibitors. Take a multivitamin to ensure you get all the vitamins and minerals you need for healthy brain function.

- Taking ten minutes out of your day for just you and you alone is a very powerful tool to combat anxiety and panic. Relax in a seated position, close your eyes, and concentrate on your breathing. Brush any negative thoughts aside. You will become hooked on this daily ritual, and it will make a difference in your life.

- Take at hot bath and be as warm and comfortable as you can. Heat pacifies the anxiety in our brains and slows us down, inside and out!

- Take a brisk walk, get on the treadmill, or pull weeds. Vigorous exercise has been proven to stop anxiety dead in its tracks.

- Try the 4-7-8 breathing technique. This tip is highly recommended. Concentrate on breathing when you feel an attack coming on. Inhale through your nose for 4 counts. Hold the breath for 7 counts. Exhale slowly through the nose for 8 counts. It is hard to be panicked when you are concentrating on your breathing.

- Prayer works. Having faith in something bigger than ourselves has gotten many people through anxiety, hysteria, and panic.

• • • •

# PINCHED NERVE

A pinched nerve can be excruciatingly painful. You should get a professional diagnosis about your pain to ensure more serious issues are not the cause. These recipes have been used throughout time and are still used today to bring relief.

## AYURVEDA: *Elderberry Syrup for Pinched Nerves*

Ayurvedic teachings use this particular method to stop pinched nerve pain and reduce inflammation and spasms. Elderberries are highly detoxifying and immune boosting. Try this recipe to ease your pain and diminish onsets of pinched nerves. Honey is also a good source of immune-boosting and anti-inflammatory properties.

**½ CUP ELDERBERRIES**

**1 CUP HONEY**

Place elderberries in a jar, cover with runny honey (or vegetable glycerin, if you prefer), and put the lid on the jar. Place in a sunny windowsill or a warm spot and leave for two weeks. If the herbs rise above the honey, you will need to press them down into the honey so they won't turn brown. After two weeks, strain and bottle. Label. Take one teaspoon up to three times a day. Store in a dark, cool area for up to six months.

## HERB: *Nerve Compress*

This herbal recipe contains herbs that have antispasmodic, analgesic, and sedative properties, to name a few. It feels good and can end that constant pain of a pinched nerve.

**1 TEASPOON ARNICA**

**1 TEASPOON ST. JOHN'S WORT**

**1 TEASPOON ELDERBERRIES**

**1 CUP BOILING WATER**

Place the herbs into the boiling water. Steep for twenty minutes; strain and discard herbs. Cool slightly, soak a washcloth in the liquid, squeeze out most of the liquid, and apply cloth to affected area for up to thirty minutes. Repeat process. Store any remainder in the refrigerator for up to forty-eight hours.

## ESSENTIAL OIL: *Godsend Nerve Rub*

The essential oils in this recipe have a multitude of warnings associated with their use. This recipe is actually one of the few times I ever use them. They are powerful, and they work well. Do a patch test (see page 4) before using this rub.

**10 DROPS BIRCH OIL**

**10 DROPS WINTERGREEN OIL**

**1 OUNCE CARRIER OIL (SUCH AS JOJOBA, SESAME, GRAPESEED, OR YOUR PREFERENCE)**

**5 DROPS VITAMIN E OIL**

Mix the ingredients in a small glass container and apply lightly to the painful area. Keep essential oil mixture away from open wounds, mucus membranes, genitals, eyes, and sensitive areas. Repeat application as needed, usually two to three times daily. Store unused portion in a glass jar with a tight-fitting lid, label it, and keep it in a cool, dark area for up to six months.

Alternating heat and ice has been a treatment used for years. The vasocon-strictor and vasodilator effects of the heat and ice help to reduce pressure on the nerve endings and stop pain. Try this old tip as a way to ease your pinched nerve pain.

Make an ice pack out of a piece of linen and some crushed ice or a bag of frozen vegetables or use an actual ice pack. Make a heat pack by filling a sock with some dry rice or dried beans and heating it in the microwave or use a hot water bottle or just a piece of linen with hot water on it. Alternate the ice pack with the heat pack and switch them out every fifteen minutes. It helps to have two packs of each so that while you are using one, you can heat or cool the other one. Repeat this ritual every hour until inflammation dissipates.

• • • •

# PLEURISY

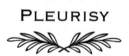

Pleurisy is an extremely painful condition that is usually caused by a viral infection in the lungs. Essential oils, herbs, Ayurveda, and home remedies abound for this ailment, but medical attention is required for quick recovery. Check with your physician to ensure these treatments will not conflict with your current medications.

In Ayurvedic treatments great healing results are achieved by placing hot packs on the chest to break up congestion and empty the lungs of fluid. There are various ways that you can make a compress heat pack.

Take a bottle filled with hot water and place it inside of a piece of linen or cotton and then place this on the chest. There are many alternatives used in the place of a hot water bottle that you can buy at your local discount store. Beads, rice, seeds, and beans are placed in various coverings to be heated in the microwave to reach a comfortable temperature to be placed on the chest. In Ayurveda heat is applied to the chest at least three times daily for twenty to forty minutes each time. In the event that the pleurisy patient has fever, then cold packs are used to replace the hot packs until fever has subsided.

## HERB: *Basil Painless Pasta*

This may sound crazy, but basil is one of the best-known pleurisy cures on the planet. You can make tea out of basil, use it in ointments, eat it just like it is, or, in this case, add plenty of it to a good dish and eat it up. This is very tasty and spicy, and the cheese helps balance out the spiciness of the basil. Use this only when you are on the mend and you can eat regular meals again.

> PASTA, ENOUGH FOR 2 SERVINGS
>
> ½ STICK BUTTER
>
> 1 TABLESPOON FLOUR (OR GLUTEN-FREE ALTERNATIVE)
>
> ¼ ONION, DICED
>
> ½ CUP BROCCOLI FLORETS
>
> 1 GARLIC CLOVE
>
> ½ CUP LIQUID STOCK
>
> ¼ CUP FRESH BASIL LEAVES, CHOPPED
>
> ¼ CUP PARMESAN CHEESE

In a large saucepan, cook pasta according to package directions. In a medium saucepan, melt butter and bring to a simmer. Add the flour and whisk while simmering for about three minutes.

Add the onion, broccoli, and garlic and lightly cook for three to five minutes. Add the liquid stock and bring to boil, then lower to simmer and cook to desired thickness.

Add the chopped basil leaves, continue cooking for one minute, and then remove from heat. Add the pasta to the sauce and sprinkle with parmesan cheese. Serve with olives, cheese, or garlic bread.

## ESSENTIAL OIL: *Pleurisy Pain Ender*

Sharp, stabbing pains are the first signs of pleurisy. You can bring relief to those pains with this essential oil inflammation and spasm fighter. Try this oil in the morning and in the evening to ease your pain and discomfort.

8 DROPS TEA TREE OIL

8 DROPS BASIL OIL

5 DROPS FRANKINCENSE OIL

4 DROPS VITAMIN E OIL

1 OUNCE CARRIER OIL (SUCH AS JOJOBA, SESAME, GRAPESEED, OR YOUR PREFERENCE)

Mix the ingredients in a small glass container and apply lightly to the area desired, such as pressure points, neck, soles of feet, temples, and chest. Keep essential oil mixture away from open wounds, mucus membranes, genitals, eyes, and sensitive areas. Repeat application as needed, usually two to three times daily. Store unused portion in a glass jar with a tight-fitting lid, label it, and keep it in a cool, dark area for up to six months.

## HOME REMEDY: *Pleurisy Tips*

There are some basic tips to follow if you find yourself suffering from pleurisy. These tips are from several different cultures around the world, so decide which works best for you.

- Use heat packs, showers, and steam to heat the chest and expel mucus from lungs.
- Do not smoke, and stay away from others who smoke.
- Stay away from spicy, heavy foods, alcohol, and caffeine.
- Take olive leaf capsules daily.
- Try to take detoxifying herbs, drink plenty of room temperature water, and keep your digestive tract clear. Getting the toxins out of your system is paramount to a speedy recovery. Fasting for two to three days is an ideal way to dry up the fluid in the lungs. After pleurisy dries, it's best to start out with goat's milk or broth for a day before progressing to solid foods.
- Get plenty of sleep. Nap when you feel like it, especially when you are in the wet/congested phase, and get all the rest you can.
- There is no better healer than plenty of vitamin D, which comes from the sun. Fresh air in your lungs and sunlight will have you feeling better in no time. After the lungs

are in the dry phase, begin slowly exercising, take walks outdoors, and do some light yoga and stretches.

- Don't take any drugs unless specified by your doctor. Try to use as few chemicals on your body as possible.

- Take a probiotic to get your gut in check. Your digestive system has a major effect on illness in the rest of your body.

- Herbal teas are full of so many healing therapeutic properties. They almost all have anti-inflammatory agents to heal and protect you where you need it most.

- Essential oils added to a salt bath help to impart healing components throughout your body and to your lungs.

• • • •

# PMS (PREMENSTRUAL SYNDROME)

Premenstrual syndrome is due to hormonal changes that take place seven to ten days before your monthly cycle. It can also affect a woman through an entire decade of menopause. These monthly changes to hormones can really affect you, your career, and your family. Try some of these recipes and tips to assuage many PMS symptoms.

### AYURVEDA: *Fiber Me Up*

In Ayurveda it is believed that the digestive system is responsible for balancing the doshas, which, when out of balance, promote disease, illness, and PMS. Balancing the doshas and flushing out the digestive tract are ways that we can get our hormones under control. Fiber-rich foods are excellent for cleaning out the digestive tract, and eating from the following list will help you achieve your goal and balance all of the doshas: almonds, avocados, black beans, blackberries, bran, broccoli, brussels sprouts, cauliflower, flaxseed, lentils, lima beans, pistachios, quinoa, raspberries, spinach, split peas, squash, strawberries, turnip greens, and wild rice. Don't forget the water—drinking ample amounts of water can flush out our systems and help us to detox.

## HERB: *Sanity Decoction*

These herbs have been used for centuries to control and balance hormones that are out of sync due to PMS. This decoction tastes great and has so many healing and soothing therapeutic properties that you will want to use it for any anxiety-producing event.

½ CUP LEMON BALM LEAVES

½ CUP ST. JOHN'S WORT

½ CUP RASPBERRY LEAF

2 CUPS BOILING WATER

Place the herbs into a mason jar. Pour the boiling water over the herbs and steep for twenty minutes or more. Strain and, if desired, add sweetener of choice. Compost or discard herbs. Drink ½–1 cup of the mixture slowly over the course of a few hours. Repeat twice daily. Remainder may be kept in a jar with a tight-fitting lid in the refrigerator for up to three days.

## ESSENTIAL OIL: *Mood-Stabilizing Spritzer*

Getting your moods and emotions under control can be the worst part of PMS. Try this spritzer with calming essential oils to help *you* be the boss of your hormones.

10 DROPS CLARY SAGE OIL

10 DROPS VETIVER OIL

10 DROPS LAVENDER OIL

5 DROPS LEMON BALM (MELISSA) OIL

1 TEASPOON WITCH HAZEL

4 OUNCES WATER

Spritzes are lighter than sprays and easier to wear on the body or in your hair. Mix the essential oils, witch hazel, and water in a spray bottle. Label. Shake well before each use. Lightly spritz the area desired, such as body, hair, clothing (check first for color damage to clothing and furniture), rooms, car, or office. The lightly scented fragrance and the healing, therapeutic properties will soon make this one of your favorite methods of using your oils. Store your spritzer in a cool, dark area for up to three months.

**HOME REMEDY:** *PMS Stress Buster*

While this may seem simple and hard to believe, this remedy is the best for PMS: learn to control your thoughts. You will be surprised how you can turn anger into happiness. Try the meditation/prayer technique below and see how breathing and thinking affect every area of your life, not just when you have PMS.

Sit in a quiet room with some low, simple music playing. Find a comfortable spot to sit where you will not be interrupted. Cross your legs and place your hands on your knees, palms up. Sit up tall and straight.

Breathe in and out fully and slowly. Concentrate on your breath. Think about all of the negative and evil thoughts going out of your body and brain with each exhale, and all of the positive, good thoughts coming in and filling you with love on each inhale.

Now practice controlling your thoughts. Your thoughts will automatically turn to negative things when you have PMS (and generally most other times as well). It is very difficult to learn to think only positive and good thoughts. The best way to do this is to start each thought with the words *thank you*.

You will be surprised at how much stress, anxiety, and tension will leave your body with this exercise. This exercise is the most important thing I do each day. You will be amazed at how a few minutes of positive thinking can affect not only your PMS but your family, your career, and your life.

· · · ·

# POISON IVY/OAK/SUMAC

Allergic reactions to these plants have been around since that first cavewoman! It's so frustratingly itchy and painful and ugly. Luckily there are many recipes that will eliminate the pain, redness, and swelling due to poison ivy, oak, or sumac—you just need to experiment to find out which one works best for you or your family.

### AYURVEDA: *Simple Ivy Treatment*

This is a simple yet effective way to treat poison ivy, oak, or sumac. There is an ingredient inside of a banana peel that will rid the site of the itch-producing acids in poison ivy. Try this the next time you get that itchy little blister!

Take the inside of a banana peel and rub it over the infected area. It will instantly stop the itch and the spread of the allergen. Repeat as often as necessary.

### HERB: *Itchy Witchy*

This simple, cheap derivative from witch hazel works so well it will seem like magic. It feels good and can abruptly stop the itch and the spread of poison ivy, oak, or sumac.

Pour a little witch hazel directly onto the area or onto a cloth or bandage and apply to the site. Leave on until liquid is evaporated. Reapply as often as five times a day until site dries up.

### ESSENTIAL OIL: *Itch Bandage*

This is a great recipe for when poison ivy first starts on your body and is contained to a small, itchy area. These essential oils contain anti-inflammatory, antifungal, and antibacterial properties to eliminate those little bumps.

2 DROPS PEPPERMINT OIL

2 DROPS SAGE OIL

½ TEASPOON CARRIER OIL (SUCH AS JOJOBA, SESAME, GRAPESEED, OR YOUR PREFERENCE)

BANDAGE

Combine the oils together in a tiny container. Apply a few drops of the mixture to the site and cover with a bandage. Reapply two or three times daily, as needed, until the infected area of skin dries out and crusts over.

### HOME REMEDY: *Poison Paste*

This is a simple recipe, and it is very common because it works. The acid neutralizer in the baking soda stops the itch and quickly begins the healing process by drying out the invasion of poison.

**1 TABLESPOON BAKING SODA**

**3 TABLESPOONS WATER**

Mix the ingredients together into a small bowl. This will form a very thick paste. Smear paste onto site of itchy bumps. Leave it on until it dries up and falls off. Reapply often or until allergen is eradicated.

• • • •

# PSORIASIS

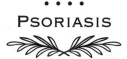

Psoriasis can be socially devastating for those suffering from it. The skin looks very inflamed, with weeping or dry wounds that spread uncontrollably. The itch that accompanies this condition is maddening. There is nothing good about psoriasis. It takes many years for most people to determine the cause. It is usually caused by allergies to a certain food or chemical. Wheat, eggs, dairy, laundry detergent, shampoo ... the list is endless. Stress often activates an outbreak of psoriasis, so try to incorporate relaxing and soothing rituals into your daily life. Psoriasis can be kept to a minimum, along with the itching, with some old techniques. The elimination diet is very useful as well. Try one of these recipes the next time a patch breaks out. Ensure with your doctor that if you are taking some sort of medication for your psoriasis, these treatments won't interfere with your current regimen.

## AYURVEDA: *Baking Soda Poultice*

In Ayurveda it is often thought that the kapha dosha is out of balance, thereby causing skin irritations and eruptions. Try following a kapha-reducing diet consisting mainly of herbs, juices, and staying away from acidic foods. Baking soda is often used in Ayurvedic treatments due to its healing properties. In this recipe the baking soda reduces itching and dries out the weeping wounds associated with psoriasis.

**¼ CUP BAKING SODA**

**1½ CUPS WARM WATER**

**GAUZE OR LINEN SQUARE**

Ensure that the water is not hot. Hot water and psoriasis do not go well together. Dissolve the baking soda into the water, stirring with a whisk. Dip a piece of gauze or linen into the mixture and apply poultice to the area affected. Leave on for ten minutes and allow site to air-dry. Heat water slightly and repeat process. Discard any remainder. Repeat entire sequence morning and night until psoriasis dries out and disappears.

## HERB: *Itch Salve*

This recipe has been handed down for many generations. We are so lucky in this day and age that the herbs we seek are just a quick trip to the local herbal shop away (or a click away on the internet). Try this psoriasis remedy for some soothing relief. Remember to keep stress reduced as much as possible, as stress aggravates psoriasis.

> 1 CUP ST. JOHN'S WORT
>
> 1 CUP CALENDULA FLOWERS
>
> 2 CUPS CARRIER OIL (SUCH AS JOJOBA, SESAME, GRAPESEED, OR YOUR PREFERENCE)
>
> 10 DROPS VITAMIN E OIL
>
> 1–2 OUNCES BEESWAX

In a saucepan pack herbs into carrier oil and cook on low for one and a half hours. Strain through cheesecloth and discard herbs. Add the vitamin E oil and 1 ounce of beeswax and stir until beeswax is melted. Pour a drop of the mixture onto the counter and run your finger through it after it has set for one minute. If it is too thick, add more carrier oil; if it is too thin, add more beeswax. Once you have the correct consistency, pour into a jar and label. Apply liberally to psoriasis areas, which may be covered lightly with gauze, if desired. Apply morning and night. Store remainder in a jar with a tight-fitting lid for up to one year.

## ESSENTIAL OIL: *Itchy Balm*

These herbs help to dry up the wounds of psoriasis and speed healing. They are also calming and can help reduce itching and inflammation.

- 1 TEASPOON BEESWAX PEARLS
- 3 TEASPOONS CARRIER OIL (SUCH AS JOJOBA, SESAME, GRAPESEED, OR YOUR PREFERENCE)
- 5 DROPS TEA TREE OIL
- 5 DROPS FRANKINCENSE OIL
- 5 DROPS LAVENDER OIL
- 4 DROPS VITAMIN E OIL

In a small pan heat the beeswax and the carrier oil on the stovetop until just melted. Pour a drop of the melted oil and wax onto the counter; check for consistency after one minute. If it is too thin, add more beeswax; if it is too thick, add more carrier oil. Add the oils to the heated mixture. Whisk lightly—it will begin hardening immediately. Pour into containers. Once cool, apply to area of outbreak. Do not apply to mucus membranes, eyes, genitals, or open wounds. Label containers and store in a dark, dry area for up to one year.

## HOME REMEDY: *Bath Ritual*

The itch-relieving and healing properties of these ingredients are known worldwide. Take a nice long comforting bath and reduce that pain and itching while healing at the same time.

- 1 CUP EPSOM SALT
- 1 TABLESPOON MINERAL OIL
- 1 TABLESPOON MILK (OPTIONAL)

Add the Epsom salt and the mineral oil to the running water. Ensure that the water is not hot, as psoriasis should never be submersed in hot water. If you add milk to the water, it will prevent the oil from floating on top of the water and sticking to your skin.

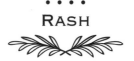

# RASH

Rashes are probably the most common form of complaint. Some rashes are from illnesses, some are from contact dermatitis, and some are from allergies. Rashes are often raised red bumpy splotches that can be located anywhere on the body. Blisters oftentimes accompany rashes. Finding out what caused the rash can be determined by your dermatologist and by just watching what chemicals you use or what foods you eat. Many alternative recipes from different cultures have been used for thousands of years to soothe and heal rashes.

### AYURVEDA: *Rash Treatment*

This recipe comes from India, where they use everyday ingredients to heal and mend ailments. Even though it is simple in ingredients and preparation, once it is applied to the skin, the paste culminates in a feeling of relief as it relieves itch and burning sensations.

1 TEASPOON CORNSTARCH

1 TEASPOON OLIVE OIL OR WATER

Mix the ingredients together in a small container until a thick paste is formed. Smear the paste mixture onto the site or onto a cloth. Do not apply to eyeballs, genitals, or open wounds. Cover with a bandage, linen, or gauze if desired. Reapply two to four times daily until rash is healed.

### HERB: *Rash Wash*

The soothing and healing properties in this wash not only feel good but will help your rash disappear! These herbs are widely known for their cicatrisant and epidermal healing effects, and they are gentle and mild to the skin.

2 TABLESPOONS CHAMOMILE FLOWERS

2 TABLESPOONS CALENDULA FLOWERS

1 CUP BOILING WATER

Place the herbs in the boiling water. Lower heat and simmer herbs for twenty minutes. Remove from heat. Strain and discard herbs. Cool the liquid to room temperature and use as a wash for the affected area. Let air-dry and repeat process three to five times daily. Discard any remainder at the end of the day.

## ESSENTIAL OIL: *Rash Ointment*

Bring glowing health to your skin with this rash soother and healer. Antiseptic, bactericidal, and moisturizing agents abound in this essential oil blend.

    1 TEASPOON BEESWAX, CHOPPED

    3 TEASPOONS CARRIER OIL (SUCH AS JOJOBA, SESAME,
        GRAPESEED, OR YOUR PREFERENCE)

    10 DROPS TEA TREE OIL

    10 DROPS NEEM OIL

    4 DROPS VITAMIN E OIL

In a small pan heat the beeswax and the carrier oil on the stovetop until just melted. Pour a drop of the melted oil and wax onto the counter and check for consistency after one minute. If it is too thin, add more beeswax; if it is too thick, add more carrier oil. Add the oils to the heated mixture. Whisk lightly; it will begin hardening immediately. Pour into containers. Once cool, apply to affected area. You may want to cover lightly with gauze to protect clothing and furniture from oils. Do not apply to mucus membranes, eyes, genitals, or open wounds. Label containers and store in a dark, dry area for up to one year.

## HOME REMEDY: *Rash Spray Away*

The healing properties in apple cider vinegar know no bounds. It is great for rashes and other skin irritations. Witch hazel is not only a great natural preservative, but it also is loaded with vitamins and minerals along with its own therapeutic properties. Keep this spray handy and use it when needed.

    1 OUNCE APPLE CIDER VINEGAR

    1 OUNCE WATER

    1 TABLESPOON WITCH HAZEL

Combine the ingredients into a spray bottle and label it. Shake well, lightly spray the rash area, and allow to air-dry. Do not spray into eyes, genitals, open wounds, or mucus membranes. Shake well before each use. Store in a cool, dark area for up to six months.

· · · ·

# RESPIRATORY INFECTION

There are many reasons for respiratory infections. Oftentimes, respiratory infections can lead to medical emergencies, which must be properly diagnosed by a physician. Ayurveda, herbs, home remedies, and essential oils have all been used for thousands of years to decrease the symptoms of infection and respiratory issues. Ensure with your medical team that any of the treatments below will not counteract any of your current medications.

### AYURVEDA: *Respiratory Milk*

This Ayurvedic recipe has tons of delicious healing properties to get you back on your feet again. Anti-inflammatory agents work to heal your lungs, throat, and sinuses and let you sleep easy.

> 1 CUP MILK
>
> 1 TEASPOON GROUND TURMERIC
>
> 1 TEASPOON HONEY

In a small saucepan, heat the milk until it just begins to boil. Remove pan from heat and stir in the turmeric and honey. Drink before bedtime.

### HERB: *Thyme Cough Syrup*

This recipe not only heals quickly but tastes good, too. This is the first herbal recipe I ever made, almost forty years ago, and it changed our lives forever by opening a world of alternative medicine to us. These decongestant, expectorant, and sudorific healing properties are little miracles.

> 1 CUP WATER
>
> ¼ CUP THYME, CHOPPED
>
> 4–6 TABLESPOONS HONEY OR SUGAR

Bring water to a boil, then add herbs and simmer for twenty-five minutes. Strain and compost or discard herbs. Add three tablespoons honey or sugar to the syrup and stir, adding more honey or sugar until it reaches desired consistency. Cool to room temperature. The standard dosage for adults is one tablespoon and for children, one teaspoon three times daily. Label and store in a tightly covered glass container in the refrigerator for up to one week.

### ESSENTIAL OIL: *Chest Reliever*

The healing properties of decongestant, sudorific, anti-inflammatory, expectorant, and analgesic properties not only relieve chest congestion, but sinus issues as well.

> 5 DROPS FRANKINCENSE OIL
>
> 5 DROPS EUCALYPTUS OIL
>
> 5 DROPS PEPPERMINT OIL
>
> 5 DROPS VITAMIN E OIL
>
> ½ OUNCE CARRIER OIL (SUCH AS JOJOBA, SESAME, GRAPESEED, OR YOUR PREFERENCE)

Mix the ingredients in a small glass container and apply lightly to the area desired, such as throat, upper back, and chest. Keep essential oil mixture away from open wounds, mucus membranes, genitals, eyes, and sensitive areas. Repeat application as needed, usually two to three times daily. Store unused portion in a glass jar with a tight-fitting lid, label it, and keep it in a cool, dark area for up to six months.

### HOME REMEDY: *Chest Poultice*

Bay leaves are renowned for their lung-healing properties. This poultice will help to break up congestion and dispel mucus. Ensure through your medical professionals that your issues are not more complicated than just congestion. This recipe is very old and has been used for centuries to break up congestion. Never use alternative medicine without first checking with your physician to make sure the treatments are compatible with your medications.

> 3–5 BAY LEAVES
>
> 1½ CUPS WATER
>
> 1 PIECE OF LINEN OR MUSLIN

Heat the bay leaves and the water on the stove until it comes to a boil. Reduce heat and simmer for twenty minutes. Remove from heat and take the bay leaves out of the water with a fork. You may place the bay leaves inside of the piece of linen or discard them. Cool the bay-infused water to room temperature. Soak the piece of linen in the water. Place linen directly onto chest, depending on the comfort of the temperature and the time of year. Leave on chest for thirty minutes or as long as it feels pleasing. Discard liquid after twenty-four hours.

· · · ·
# RESTLESS LEG SYNDROME

This ailment is a very hard to describe feeling experienced by people, from an occasional incident of restless leg syndrome to having an episode hundreds of times a night. RLS, while difficult to explain to others, may cause chronic sleep deprivation. Imagine waking up hundreds of times a night as soon as your brain drifts off to sleep—and it often happens until the early morning hours. Night after night. Year after year. Many studies point to a lack of vitamins, specifically iron, zinc, and magnesium, which is easily correctable by taking those vitamins. Essential oils, home remedies, Ayurveda, and herbs have all been used to bring relief to the vibrating, muscle-stretching legs of a person suffering from RLS.

### AYURVEDA: *Ayurvedic Leg Massage*

In Ayurveda the vata constitution imbalance is primarily diagnosed as the reason for RLS. Treating the vata to reduce it is the best way for long-term riddance of RLS. An effective treatment nightly is the vata-reducing and grounding benefits of sesame oil.

Warm one tablespoon sesame oil by rubbing it briskly between the palms of your hands. Slowly rub the oil onto the legs, below the knees, and the feet. Massage the sesame oil deeply into your skin and between your toes. The warming, soothing action of the sesame oil helps you get a good night's sleep and lowers the vata, thereby balancing out the doshas. Ensure that you have an old sheet or covering on your bed so that you don't mind it being stained by the oil.

## HERB: *Restless Leg Syndrome Wash*

Many people have had success with this wash. The herbal therapeutic properties help you to reach a level of sleep that cannot be disturbed by RLS. This soothing wash should be applied directly before bedtime.

1 CUP WATER

2 TABLESPOONS ST. JOHN'S WORT

2 TABLESPOONS ROMAN CHAMOMILE FLOWERS

Bring water to a boil, then add herbs. Remove from heat, cover, and steep for ten to fifteen minutes. Strain and cool until desired temperature for skin application is reached. Discard herbs. Dip a square of linen into the wash and apply to lower legs and feet. Allow mixture to air-dry onto your skin. Discard remainder of liquid.

## ESSENTIAL OIL: *Restless Leg Syndrome Rub*

This recipe contains essential oils that calm the mind, relieve the nerves, and help produce a good night's sleep with its sedative and tranquilizing properties.

5 DROPS FRANKINCENSE OIL

5 DROPS MARJORAM OIL

5 DROPS VALERIAN ROOT OIL

5 DROPS VITAMIN E

1 OUNCE CARRIER OIL (SUCH AS JOJOBA, SESAME, GRAPESEED, OR YOUR PREFERENCE)

Mix the ingredients in a small glass container and apply lightly to the area desired, such as feet, calves, thighs, or lower back. Protect furniture and clothing from stains by wearing an old T-shirt or using an old sheet on the bed. Keep essential oil mixture away from open wounds, mucus membranes, genitals, eyes, and sensitive areas. Repeat application as needed. Store unused portion in a glass jar with a tight-fitting lid, label it, and keep it in a cool, dark area for up to six months.

There are home remedies for everything, and RLS is no different. Here are the best-known tips that have helped thousands of people in the past, and one of these tips may just be the one that you are looking for to get rid of RLS once and for all.

- No alcohol, sugar, or caffeine.

- Alternate warm and cool packs on your legs for thirty minutes before bedtime.

- Up your intake of iron, zinc, and magnesium. This cure worked for me.

- Exercise—specifically, more walking. Try getting a good walk in every night after your evening meal.

- Sexual release.

- Leg massages. You can do these yourself and use oils that you like to promote sleep.

- Stretching the leg muscles seems to work at ending RLS in many people. Try some long, lean yoga poses: forward bends, tree, mountain, and simple stretches.

- Ivory soap slivers in your socks, worn to bed. I have never tried this, but many people swear by it.

- Eat light at supper, and no snacking afterward.

· · · ·

# RINGWORM

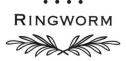

Ringworm is actually not a worm, but a fungus. It is contagious and can be treated effectively by medications available today from your doctor. For centuries ringworm was cured by herbs, Ayurveda, home remedies, and essential oils. When first caught, ringworm can be relatively easy to eliminate, but once it starts spreading over the entire body, it is much harder to eradicate.

## AYURVEDA: *Ringworm Bandage*

This old Ayurvedic recipe uses turmeric, one of the greatest anti-inflammatory agents on earth. The itching, redness, and bumpiness will dissipate, and the viral fungus will die. Repeat as needed.

**½ TEASPOON TURMERIC POWDER**

**½ TEASPOON COCONUT OIL**

Mix and blend the ingredients together in a small container until a thick paste is formed. Smear the paste mixture onto the ringworm or onto cloth. Cover with a bandage, linen, or gauze, if desired, and tape in place. Apply two to four times daily until fungus is healed. Reapply for one week or more if signs of ringworm are present. Store any remainder in a jar with a tight-fitting lid for up to forty-eight hours.

## HERB: *Ringworm Paste*

Garlic kills fungus. Try this ancient herbal remedy to banish that ringworm from your life and to keep it from spreading all over your body. The antifungal properties in garlic and honey will eliminate this contagious virus before it spreads.

**1 GARLIC CLOVE, MINCED**

**1 TEASPOON HONEY**

**1 TEASPOON COCONUT OR SESAME OIL**

Mix and mash the ingredients together in a small container until a thick paste is formed. Smear the paste mixture onto the site or onto cloth. Cover with a bandage, linen, or gauze, if desired, and tape to keep in place. Apply two to four times daily until ringworm is healed. I often reapply for a few days after any sign of the ringworm is present in order to make sure it is all gone. Store any remainder in a jar with a tight-fitting lid for up to forty-eight hours.

## ESSENTIAL OIL: *Ringworm Fighter*

The antifungal ingredients in these oils work with antimicrobial, antibacterial, and fungicidal healing properties to kill that ringworm and banish it from your body.

1 DROP TEA TREE OIL

1 DROP LAVENDER OIL

1 DROP LEMON OIL

½ TEASPOON CARRIER OIL (SUCH AS JOJOBA, SESAME, GRAPESEED, OR YOUR PREFERENCE)

Mix the ingredients well in a very small container. Apply a few drops of the mixture to a bandage or a piece of gauze with a cotton swab and secure to site. Leave on all day or overnight. Repeat process for up to one week. Label and store remainder in a small jar with a tight-fitting lid. Store in a cool, dark area for up to two weeks.

HOME REMEDY: *Worm Wash*

This centuries-old wash remedy is a favorite of many grandmothers and is as old as time. It's simple, effective, and loaded with so many healing properties—and it doesn't burn or sting. When applied properly, apple cider vinegar is a powerful antifungal medicine.

½ CUP APPLE CIDER VINEGAR

½ CUP WATER

Combine ingredients into a bowl and stir with a spoon or whisk. Dip a soft washcloth into the blend, apply the mixture to the ringworm, and let air-dry. Keep on area as long as comfortable, from fifteen to thirty minutes, rewetting as needed. Repeat process several times a day for seven to ten days. Never apply to open wounds, eyeballs, genitals, or near sensitive body parts. Store remainder in the refrigerator for up to forty-eight hours.

• • • •

# SCARS

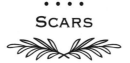

The fibrous tissue that forms when the body is healing itself is a scar. Usually scars don't bother us and are a reminder of a past event. But occasionally a scar may form on the face or is the type of scar that leaves us with reminders of something we wish to forget. It is nice to know that scars can be reduced drastically by using home remedies, herbs, Ayurveda, or some type of safe alternative healing. It takes a while for the agents to work on the scar, so remain faithful to the routine you choose, and you could see amazing results.

## AYURVEDA: *Ayurvedic Scar Paste*

Two of the most natural healing elements on earth are lemon and honey; we use them for coughs, colds, viruses, and a host of other issues. But did you know that honey and lemon also have great cicatrisant and vulnerary properties for your skin? Try this recipe every day for a couple of weeks and watch your scars slowly recede in color and toughness.

4 DROPS LEMON JUICE

4 DROPS HONEY

Mix the ingredients well in a very small container. Apply a few drops of the mixture to a bandage or a piece of gauze and secure to site (with tape if using gauze). Leave on for several hours or overnight. Discard any remainder.

## HERB: *Herbal Scar Oil*

Calendula oil has anti-inflammatory, vulnerary, and skin-smoothing properties to take that scar from annoying to nonexistent. Making your own calendula oil out of pretty marigold flowers is an overwhelmingly powerful feeling of accomplishment. Calendula flowers are readily available as pot marigold. You can purchase them online already picked, bagged, and waiting for you to use as skin-softening agents.

1½ CUPS CARRIER OIL (SUCH AS JOJOBA, SESAME, GRAPESEED, OR YOUR PREFERENCE)

1 CUP CALENDULA FLOWERS, FINELY CHOPPED

½ TEASPOON VITAMIN E OIL

Pour carrier oil into a small crockpot. Add calendula flowers and stir. Put lid on crockpot and turn on low for eight hours. Cool completely. Strain through cheesecloth and discard herbs. Add the vitamin E oil, bottle, and label. Apply to scarred skin morning and night until scar is greatly diminished. Store remainder in a cool, dark area for up to one year.

## ESSENTIAL OIL: *Rosehip Scar Rub*

Rosehip seed oil has been used since before the days of Cleopatra to remove and diminish scars. Rosehip contains vulnerary, anti-inflammatory, astringent, and cicatrisant properties to help with tough skin issues.

**15 DROPS ROSEHIP SEED OIL**

**5 DROPS VITAMIN E OIL**

**½ OUNCE CARRIER OIL (SUCH AS JOJOBA, SESAME, GRAPESEED, OR YOUR PREFERENCE)**

Mix the ingredients in a small glass container and apply lightly to the area of the scar. Protect furniture and clothing from stains by wearing old clothing. Keep essential oil mixture away from open wounds, mucus membranes, genitals, eyes, and sensitive areas. Repeat application as needed, usually two times daily. Store unused portion in a glass jar with a tight-fitting lid, label it, and keep it in a cool, dark area for up to six months.

## HOME REMEDY: *Scar Smear*

A smear of many household products can work well in reducing the signs and appearance of scars. Try dabbing a few drops of these ground-up or blended ingredients onto your scar or onto a bandage and cover your scar for a day. Repeat process daily for two weeks. Try one or try them all to see which one works best for you.

**GROUND POTATO**

**GROUND GINGER**

**GROUND CUCUMBER**

**GROUND GARLIC**

**GROUND ALMONDS AND WATER**

**ALOE VERA**

Mix a half teaspoon ingredient with one-fourth teaspoon olive oil or water or put on straight. Apply to scar, cover with bandage, and leave for several hours or overnight. Discard remainder.

• • • •

# SLEEP APNEA

Sleep apnea is responsible for causing an untold number of people annually to lose copious amounts of sleep each night, and they usually don't even know it. People wake from tens to hundreds of times a night due to breathing interruptions and then fall back to sleep, only to repeat the same pattern minutes or seconds later. New medications and machines are available now to help with sleep apnea, but home remedies, Ayurveda, essential oils, and herbal remedies have abounded forever in helping a person have uninterrupted sleep without breathing interruptions. Ensure with your doctor that these remedies won't interfere with your current medications.

## AYURVEDA: *Sleep Paste*

This is the recipe used in India to relieve breathing during the night. Try this simple remedy the next time you notice your loved one or yourself waking up repeatedly. Apply nightly for best results.

⅛ TEASPOON POWDERED NUTMEG

⅛ TEASPOON GHEE

Mix the ingredients together in a spoon before bedtime. Using your fingertips, apply to the upper cheekbone and eyebrow area. Use caution and do not get near or in the eyes. Allow to dry on face and sleep with mixture on face. Discard any remainder.

## HERB: *Breathe Deep Tea*

This tea has the lung-expanding, sleep-inducing, airway-opening properties to help you overcome nighttime sleep apnea issues. Drink a cup nightly before bed to reduce your chances of waking up all night due to breathing issues. Sudorific, tranquilizing, decongestant, and expectorant properties work together to give you a peaceful night of good sleep.

1 CUP WATER

½ TEASPOON VALERIAN ROOT, CHOPPED

½ TEASPOON CHAMOMILE

1 PINCH POWDERED NUTMEG

Bring water to a boil, then add herbs. Remove from heat, cover, and steep for six to eight minutes. Strain and, if desired, add sweetener of choice. Compost or discard herbs.

## ESSENTIAL OIL: *Super Respiratory Sleeping Salve*

The sudorific and tranquilizing properties in this salve help to keep you sleeping soundly. The decongestant and expectorant properties help you to breathe properly all night long.

1 TEASPOON BEESWAX

1 OUNCE CARRIER OIL (SUCH AS JOJOBA, SESAME, GRAPESEED, OR YOUR PREFERENCE)

8 DROPS LAVENDER OIL

7 DROPS PEPPERMINT OIL

6 DROPS ROMAN CHAMOMILE OIL

6 DROPS EUCALYPTUS OIL

5 DROPS THYME OIL

4 DROPS TEA TREE OIL

4 DROPS VITAMIN E OIL

In a small pan heat the beeswax and carrier oil on the stovetop until just melted. Pour a drop of the melted oil and wax onto the counter and check for consistency after one minute. If it is too thin, add more beeswax; if it is too thick, add more carrier oil. Add the oils to the heated mixture. Whisk lightly, and it will begin hardening immediately. Pour into containers. Once cool, apply to chest, neck, or upper back. Do not apply to mucus membranes, eyes, genitals, or open wounds. Label containers and store in a dark, dry area for up to one year.

HOME REMEDY: *Breathing Technique*

Working on your breathing techniques any time of the day, but especially at night, can work wonders for your sleep apnea issues. Try breathing exercises before bed and notice the peaceful night's sleep you are bound to enjoy.

Sit in a comfortable chair or on a rug or carpeted floor.

Sit up straight with your shoulders back, thereby expanding your lungs. Cross your legs, resting your palms, face up, on your knees.

Begin by breathing long, slow, even, deep breaths. Repeat for ten breaths.

Relax. Begin to push yourself when breathing out by going two to four seconds longer on the exhales.

Begin holding your breath for four counts between inhales and exhales.

You are now inhaling for four counts, holding your breath for four counts, and exhaling for six to eight counts. Complete this process for ten breaths.

Cover one of your nostrils by pinching it lightly with your thumb. Inhale and exhale deeply for ten counts through one nostril, then repeat with the other nostril.

Finish by letting yourself fall into a regular breathing pattern. You should feel very relaxed and your lungs will feel light and airy. Good night!

• • • •

# SMELL, LOSS OF (ANOSMIA)

Losing your sense of smell can be devastating. You worry about burning smells, body odor, and the loss of beauty in the smell of flowers, baby powder, or hot chocolate cake. Regaining one's sense of smell is not a hopeless endeavor. Home remedies, essential oils, herbs, and Ayurvedic practices offer numerous ways in which people have reclaimed that lost sense.

AYURVEDA: *Zinc Aroma*

In Ayurvedic practice it is believed that zinc is the culprit in losing the sense of smell. You can take zinc supplements or you can fill yourself with rich, satisfying zinc-containing foods. The following list of foods will provide you with an idea of what and how you should be eating to regain that lost sense:

brown rice, cashews, chickpeas, flaxseed, garlic, kidney beans, lima beans, oysters, peanuts, peas, pumpkin seeds, salmon, sesame seeds, shrimp, spinach, squash seeds, watermelon seeds, and wheat germ.

### HERB: *Aroma Tea*

This is the recipe for an age-old drink that has been reported to bring back the sense of smell. While drinking this tea, hold the cup close to your nostrils and breathe deeply in through your nose between drinks.

**1 CUP WATER**

**½ TEASPOON THYME LEAVES**

**½ TEASPOON CALENDULA FLOWERS**

**½ TEASPOON LAVENDER FLOWERS**

Bring water to a boil, then add herbs. Remove from heat, cover, and steep for six to eight minutes. Strain and, if desired, add sweetener of choice. Compost or discard herbs.

### ESSENTIAL OIL: *Peppermint Steam Inhalation*

Smelling peppermint has long been thought to bring back the sense of smell. This is an excellent way to get the peppermint steam into your nostrils and brain. This is not a remedy for children, as the boiling water may scald them.

**13 DROPS PEPPERMINT OIL**

**2 CUPS BOILING WATER**

Pour boiling water into a bowl or a pan. Drop the essential oils into the boiling water. Place a towel over your head while holding your head about 12–18 inches over the steaming bowl. Make sure the towel covers all sides of your head, draping down and covering the sides of the bowl, allowing none of the steam to escape. Breathe into the steam deeply through your nostrils for as long as you can do it or until the water no longer steams. Discard any remaining liquid.

## HOME REMEDY: *Smell-Inducing Home Remedy*

Rumors abound over this recommended remedy for anosmia. During research when asking others what they have heard works, this is the recipe I was told the most. Everyone stated that this was rumored to work on the first few tries. If I ever lose my sense of smell, this will be the first recipe I use to restore it.

### 2 DROPS CASTOR OIL

Dip your finger into the castor oil and, tilting your head back, allow one drop to enter your nostril. Repeat on opposite side. Use a cotton swab to rub the oil around the interior of the nostrils and leave for remainder of the day. Repeat process daily until smell is back and odors are received again.

• • • •

## SNORING

A lot of resentment can build up in the person who shares their bed with a snorer. After medical intervention does not provide a cure, people often turn to home remedies or alternative treatments to stop snoring and bring harmony back into the household. One of these recipes may be able to help you to regain a peaceful night's sleep.

## AYURVEDA: *Snorer's Ghee*

Placing certain ingredients inside the nostrils can help tremendously with ending snoring once and for all. This old Ayurvedic ghee remedy is cheap and easy to make and use. Practicing dosha balancing can also help relieve snoring. Gargle with half sesame oil and half water to reduce vata (spit it all out), which is responsible for moving air through the body.

Making ghee is easy, resourceful, and fun. Ghee is very healthy to cook with in place of butter or oil and is useful in many Ayurvedic recipes. Take a pound of pure, real grass-fed butter (grass-fed has more nutrient value) and cook it on low on top of the stove on very, very low heat. Do not stir. All of the sediment will stick to the bottom of the pan. Cook for about thirty minutes and don't stir it. Remove foam from top as needed. When the butter looks like pure liquid gold on top, with the dark brown pieces stuck to the bottom of the pan, gently remove from heat. Through a coffee filter or fine cheesecloth, slowly strain the ghee into a glass bowl with a tight-fitting lid. Discard brown sediment. The ghee may be stored at room temperature for up to one year. To treat snoring, gently dip into cooled ghee with a cotton swab and rub the inside of each nostril with a few drops. Sleep well!

### HERB: *Snorer's Herbal Tea*

Drinking this herbal tea blend an hour before bedtime can help the snorer due to all of the respiratory healing properties in these herbs. Nettle and thyme are both such healing, relaxing, and decongesting herbs.

> 1 CUP WATER
>
> 1 TEASPOON NETTLE LEAVES
>
> 1 TEASPOON THYME LEAVES

Bring water to a boil, then add herbs. Remove from heat, cover, and steep for six to eight minutes. Strain and, if desired, add sweetener of choice. Compost or discard herbs.

### ESSENTIAL OIL: *Snoring Diffuser Blend*

These essential oils have long been used to open breathing passages and allow for a snorer to breathe through the nose instead of the mouth. With all of the diffusers available today, it's easy to run this blend at night and experiment with what oils work for your family.

> 5 DROPS PEPPERMINT OIL
>
> 5 DROPS EUCALYPTUS OIL
>
> WATER

Add oils and water to diffuser and run as desired.

### HOME REMEDY: *Garlic Snoring Cure*

Garlic has many qualities that will help reduce inflammation and help with respiratory issues. Garlic is a natural all-around healer for a million complaints. Many snorers swear by this remedy, and it has been used for thousands of years: chew a clove of garlic before bedtime and the slight swelling in your throat will relax and make sleeping easier and safer.

· · · ·
## SORE THROAT

When experiencing a sore throat, I often think how easy it is to take swallowing for granted. The pain is unbearable and makes talking and sleeping a whole new experience in misery. A sore throat fatigues our bodies and minds from the constant pain. Many remedies have been used for ages to put an end to the pain that accompanies a sore throat.

### AYURVEDA: *Throat Gargle*

Gargling for a sore throat is an age-old practice, and this is a gargle recipe that has been handed down in Ayurvedic medicine for thousands of years. Anti-inflammatory, antiviral, and antibiotic agents work together to bring rapid relief. In Ayurveda a sore throat could be caused by an excess of vata. Balance your doshas by eating cooked root vegetables and doing the yoga mountain pose.

1 CUP WATER

1 TEASPOON SAGE LEAVES

1 TEASPOON TURMERIC

1 TEASPOON HONEY

Bring water to a boil, then add sage. Cook on very low heat for about ten minutes or until the water is dissipated by half. Remove from heat, cover, and steep for ten to twenty minutes. Strain and compost or discard herbs. Stir in turmeric and honey. Cool slightly. When ready, take one tablespoon into your mouth and gargle as far back into your throat as is comfortable. Do not swallow; spit it out. Repeat several times daily. Remainder may be kept in refrigerator for up to three days.

### HERB: *Throat Decoction*

Marshmallow root contains the anti-inflammatory and healing properties to bring quick and effective relief to your sore throat. Take this blend throughout the day and you will feel much better by bedtime!

⅓ CUP MARSHMALLOW ROOT, CHOPPED

¾ QUART WATER

CINNAMON (OPTIONAL)

1 TABLESPOON HONEY (OPTIONAL)

Place the chopped marshmallow root into a mason jar. Pour boiling water over the herbs. Allow the herbs to steep for twenty to forty-five minutes, covered. Strain the mixture and compost or discard the herbs. Add honey and cinnamon if desired. Cool. Drink one-third of the mixture slowly over the course of a few hours. Repeat twice daily until desired results are achieved. Remainder may be kept in a jar with a tight-fitting lid in the refrigerator for up to three days.

## ESSENTIAL OIL: *Anti-Inflammatory Rub*

This essential oil blend contains powerful anti-inflammatory properties to reduce swelling and fight infection. This is my go-to rub in the fall when I seem to get a sore throat regularly.

10 DROPS PEPPERMINT OIL

10 DROPS TEA TREE OIL

5 DROPS SAGE OIL

5 DROPS BERGAMOT OIL

5 DROPS VITAMIN E OIL

1 OUNCE CARRIER OIL (SUCH AS JOJOBA, SESAME, GRAPESEED, OR YOUR PREFERENCE)

Mix the ingredients in a small glass container and apply lightly to the area desired, such as pressure points, neck, soles of feet, temples, and chest. Keep essential oil mixture away from open wounds, mucus membranes, genitals, eyes, and sensitive areas. Repeat application as needed, usually two to three times daily. Store unused portion in a glass jar with a tight-fitting lid, label it, and keep it in a cool, dark area for up to six months.

## HOME REMEDY: *Sore Throat Sip*

This sure does do the trick of relieving a sore throat. Honey and apple cider vinegar are both extremely healing and loaded with therapeutic properties that work well in combination to rid you of that pain.

¼ CUP WATER

1 TABLESPOON APPLE CIDER VINEGAR

1 TABLESPOON HONEY

Blend all of the ingredients into a jar that has a tight-fitting lid. Take one teaspoon of the mixture by mouth up to four times daily for immediate relief. Store remainder, covered, in refrigerator for up to three days. Ensure that you stir or shake before each dosage as the honey will settle at the bottom.

• • • •

# SPLINTER

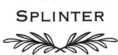

That tiny foreign material that buries itself under your skin can lead to some really annoying pain. If you let it fester, then an infection will set in, and it's like a domino effect of pain and regret. Get rid of the splinter easily and quickly by using one of these remedies to remove it.

## AYURVEDA: *Ayurvedic Drawing Paste*

Onions have been used for centuries to remove a splinter in Ayurvedic traditions. A fresh onion with lots of juice in it works best. This simple remedy with a common household item is quick and easy.

Slice an onion very thin. Take one of the slices and mash it up in a bowl with a fork. When it is a juicy, lumpy mess, apply a dab of the concoction to a bandage or a piece of linen. Affix the bandage to the splinter site and leave on for a few hours or overnight. Once the bandage is removed, grasp the splinter with tweezers and pull out.

## HERB: *Comfort Me, Comfrey*

Drawing out a splinter is just one of the ways this herbal vulnerary is used. Make up a jar of this ointment and you will have it on hand for all types of wounds, injuries, and needs, including to draw out splinters and avoid infection.

1 CUP OLIVE OIL

½ CUP COMFREY ROOT, CHOPPED

1 OUNCE BEESWAX

8 DROPS VITAMIN E OIL

Place the oil and the comfrey in a pan and cook on very, very low heat in oven for one to three hours or on extremely low heat on stovetop. Strain and discard herbs. Add beeswax and the vitamin E oil, letting the beeswax melt as you stir the blend. Pour mixture into a jar with a tight-fitting lid and label it. Apply to splinter and cover with a bandage for a few hours or overnight. When bandage is removed, grasp the splinter and pull it out. Remainder may be stored in a cool, dark area for up to one year.

## ESSENTIAL OIL: *Oil Splinter Remover*

These essential oils have been used forever for their drawing power and ability to easily draw a splinter from the skin. I have used this method in the past and had great success with it.

1 DROP FRANKINCENSE OIL

1 DROP TEA TREE OIL

BANDAGE

Apply the drops of the mixture to a bandage or a piece of gauze and secure to splinter site. Leave on for several hours or overnight. Using tweezers, grasp the edge of the splinter that has started coming out, and pull at the same angle that the splinter is laying.

## HOME REMEDY: *Easy Splinter Paste*

This old home remedy has withstood the test of time. It's painless and works wonders on drawing out splinters.

**1 TEASPOON BAKING SODA**

**¼ TEASPOON WATER**

Mix the ingredients well in a very small container. More water may be added if mixture is too thick. Apply a few drops of the mixture to a bandage or a piece of gauze and secure to splinter site. Leave on for several hours or overnight. Once bandage is removed, pull splinter out using tweezers. Store remainder in a small jar with a tight-fitting lid. Store in a cool, dark area for up to two weeks.

· · · ·

# STRESS

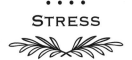

Stress is one of the major contributors to disease and illness. In our fast-paced society, it's easy to become overwhelmed by even simple everyday tasks. Herbs, essential oils, Ayurveda, and home remedies abound to teach us how to reduce stress, or at least to handle it in a way that the stress won't make us ill.

## AYURVEDA: *Stress Morning Drink*

In Ayurvedic remedies it is believed that too much stress puts the body through too many chemical reactions, and stress should be reduced before you begin each day. Besides waking up and performing cleaning rituals such as showering, grooming, self-oil massage, and yoga, Ayurvedic practitioners also begin the day with a morning drink to reduce stress for the day ahead.

**1 CUP MILK**

**⅛ TEASPOON CARDAMOM**

**⅛ TEASPOON NUTMEG**

Heat the milk on low until warm. Add the cardamom and nutmeg and any sweetener desired. Drink slowly while planning your peaceful, stress-free day.

## HERB: *Zen Tea*

Of all the herbal and relaxing teas that I like to drink for different reasons, this recipe will always live up to its name and take me to a place of peace. These herbs help to relieve stress and get rid of those negative thoughts.

> 1 CUP WATER
>
> 1 TEASPOON CHAMOMILE FLOWERS
>
> 1 TEASPOON ST. JOHN'S WORT
>
> 1 TEASPOON HONEY (OPTIONAL)

Bring water to a boil, then add herbs. Remove from heat, cover, and steep for six to eight minutes. Strain and, if desired, add sweetener of choice. Compost or discard herbs. Drink and let those feelings of relaxation overtake your mind.

## ESSENTIAL OIL: *Happy Oil Spray*

The list of essential oils that reduce the stress-induced chemical reactions in our bodies is very long. A few of these oils are basil, benzoin, cardamom, chamomile, cypress, lavender, lemon, lemon balm (*Melissa*), patchouli, peppermint, petitgrain, rose, spikenard, and ylang-ylang. You can use any of these oils, and a host of others, to make this spray. Use it on yourself, your car, your office, or anywhere that you need to have a calming Zen moment for yourself. It works on others around you that are stressed, too. You can help them calm down, and they won't even realize that aromatherapy is at work!

> 10 DROPS BERGAMOT OIL
>
> 8 DROPS NEROLI OIL
>
> 6 DROPS CASSIA OIL
>
> 4 DROPS HELICHRYSUM OIL
>
> 4 OUNCES WATER
>
> 1 TEASPOON WITCH HAZEL

Add all ingredients to a dark-colored spray bottle to prevent sunlight from damaging contents. Shake bottle before you spray. Do not spray into open wounds, genitals, eyes, or mucus membranes. Store in a cool, dark area for up to three months. Shake well before each use to combine the ingredients.

## HOME REMEDY: *Natural Stress Reducers*

We've heard all of these before, but actually putting these tips into practice is what works. Sometimes, these rituals feel like all you have to cling to in times of stress. You will love having these techniques at your fingertips at a moment's notice. You can avoid stress by incorporating some of these exercises daily, and that is the best news of all.

- Yoga's corpse pose is one of the most relaxing and stress-reducing asanas I've ever performed. Anyone can do it. Lie on a flat, comfortable surface. Rest your arms by your sides, palms up. Let your feet fall where they may. Then just close your eyes and breathe. It's that easy. Try it for three minutes and watch your stress evaporate.

- Eat a healthy diet full of fruits and vegetables. Try juicing, vegetarian, and other healthy diet practices to get all of the good nutrition, vitamins, and minerals that control those brain chemicals.

- Walking not only strengthens our bodies, but being in nature gives us a strong sense of peace, and the sun provides us with vitamin D. Take a hike for stress!

- You will be hard pressed to find a more reliable source of stress relief than meditation. Relax in a seated position; close your eyes; place your hands, palms up, on knees; and concentrate on your breathing. Banish any negative thoughts and return your thoughts to your breathing. You will become hooked on this daily ritual, and it will make a major difference in your life.

- Salt baths provide such soothing and relaxing components. You cannot be stressed when you are soaking in a tub of heaven!

- Try diffusing some essential oils that are well known for their calming therapeutic properties, such as lavender, melissa, clary sage, vetiver, and lemon.

- Prayer and gratitude are the ultimate stress reducers and my number-one favorite calming method. Try writing down ten things you are grateful for. It really works and will rewire your brain.

• • • •
# STYE (EYE)

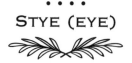

This annoying little bump—which usually appears on the eyelid or lash line for no apparent reason—is itchy and painful. It is usually caused by an infected sweat gland. Sties have been treated for thousands of years with various natural healing recipes. Try one or two of these and get some quick relief from that "sticker in my eye" feeling.

## AYURVEDA: *Eye Tea*

In India green tea is the tea of choice, and they have many uses for those tea bags after they drink it. Treating a stye with the used green tea bag is normal practice in Ayurvedic care and treatment and is simple but effective.

Close the eyes and place a wet green tea bag over the stye. Relax in this position for as long as comfortable, up to ten minutes. Repeat process several times a day until stye is eradicated.

## HERB: *Raspberry Stye Linen*

This herbal recipe has been handed down for generations. Raspberry leaf is loaded with anti-inflammatory and astringent properties to heal and soothe the stye.

2 CUPS WATER

½ CUP RASPBERRY LEAF

LINEN OR GAUZE

Bring water to a boil, then add herbs. Remove from heat, cover, and steep for ten to twenty minutes. Strain. Compost or discard herbs. Cool liquid to room temperature. Dip a piece of linen or gauze into the mixture and wring out slightly. Lay poultice over closed eye and rest for ten minutes. Repeat three or four times throughout the day. Remainder may be kept in refrigerator, in a container with a tight-fitting lid, for up to twenty-four hours.

## ESSENTIAL OIL: *Tea Tree Stye Relief*

The anti-inflammatory ingredients in tea tree oil will shrink that stye and have you blinking like normal in no time.

Using a cotton swab lightly dipped in tea tree oil, softly go around the outer eye area, the outer orbital socket, with the oil. Do not place the oil directly onto the lash line or eyeball. The therapeutic properties will work at the cellular level to absorb and disperse the anti-inflammatory agents to the inflamed part of the eye. Never place any essential oils onto or near the eyeball but allow oil to soak into the outer eye area. Repeat process daily until stye is gone.

## HOME REMEDY: *Potato Stye Press*

This is a very old home remedy and no one seems to know quite how it works, but it has worked wonderfully for thousands of people over the course of time. If you have a potato in your kitchen, why not give it a try?

### 1 TEASPOON GRATED POTATO

Mince and grind the potato into a paste. Apply the wet potato to the stye, being careful to not get it into the actual eyeball. Hold potato on stye with fingertips or bandage for as long as possible. It can reduce the swelling almost immediately. Repeat process twice daily for one week or until stye is gone.

• • • •

# SUNBURN

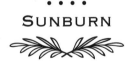

Who hasn't had a sunburn? It doesn't hurt while you are getting it, but later in the day—*ouch*! There are tons of alternative remedies for sunburns, and you probably have most of the pain-relieving cures in your own home. Herbs, essential oils, home remedies, and Ayurvedic treatments are cost effective, yet they work as good as the sunburn treatments on the market today.

## AYURVEDA: *Cucumber Paste*

This Ayurvedic remedy is easy to make and so cooling. The febrifuge properties will pull that fever right out of the skin. This sounds so good you may want to eat it, but don't; just rub it on and heal that burn!

½ CUCUMBER, PEELED AND DICED

¼ CUP PLAIN YOGURT

Mash cucumber into a paste and blend with yogurt. Rub paste on sunburned areas and allow to remain as long as is comfortable or for ten to twenty minutes, then rinse off. Repeat process twice daily. Store remainder of mixture in refrigerator for up to forty-eight hours.

## HERB: *Sunburn Spray*

Plantain has been used for sunburn for centuries, as has apple cider vinegar. Combining plantain and ACV together is a powerhouse cure for a sunburn. This spray cools, relieves pain, and heals the skin as it soaks in.

1 CUP WATER

2 TABLESPOONS PLANTAIN LEAVES

3 TABLESPOONS APPLE CIDER VINEGAR

Bring water to a boil, then add plantain. Remove from heat, cover, and steep for twenty minutes. Strain. Compost or discard herbs. Cool the liquid and add the apple cider vinegar. Pour into a spray bottle and spray the sunburned area. Repeat three times daily until sunburn is gone. If you do not have a spray bottle, you can make a wash and use linen to apply as a compress to the skin. Store remainder in a cool area for up to one month.

## ESSENTIAL OIL: *Burn Spray*

This recipe contains cooling, skin-soothing, redness-reducing properties to bring that sunburn heat down as well as analgesic properties to reduce the pain. Febrifuge agents help to take the heat out and reduce any surface fever.

20 DROPS PEPPERMINT OIL

10 DROPS LAVENDER OIL

10 DROPS TEA TREE OIL

2 TABLESPOONS WITCH HAZEL

3½ OUNCES WATER

Add all ingredients to a dark-colored spray bottle to prevent sunlight from damaging contents. Shake bottle and spray onto sunburned areas of skin. Do not spray into open wounds, genitals, eyes, or mucus membranes. Store in a cool, dark area for up to three months. Shake well before each use to combine the ingredients.

**HOME REMEDY:** *Suck Out the Heat Bath*

Many home remedies for sunburn relief include a tepid bath with ingredients that treat sunburns by cooling, containing emollient, febrifuge, and anti-inflammatory agents. Try one of these remedies the next time you have too much fun in the sun. These healing products are already in your home!

½ CUP APPLE CIDER VINEGAR

or

½ CUP MILK

or

½ CUP BAKING SODA

or

½ CUP ALOE VERA GEL

or

¼ CUP HONEY

Relax in a tepid tub of water that has one of these ingredients included. Stay in the tub as long as the water is comfortable.

· · · ·
# TENDONITIS

Tendonitis pain occurs when the tendons become inflamed and make it almost impossible to complete any task requiring that part of the body. Medical breakthroughs in surgery have been proven to work in the last couple of decades. If you are not up to having surgery yet, these essential oil, home remedy, herbal and Ayurvedic recipes can give you relief from the pain and suffering of tendonitis.

## AYURVEDA: *Tendonitis Dosha Balance*

When the doshas (vata, kapha, pitta) are out of balance, they produce illness. When tendonitis is the ailment, then pitta is more than likely the culprit that needs reducing. Follow these recommendations to bring that pitta back into check.

- Take a stroll or meditate in the moonlight.
- Don't eat hard cheeses, nuts, grapefruits, or lemons.
- Do eat berries, green leafy vegetables, basmati rice, chicken, and milk.
- Drink ginseng or sage tea.
- Take a cool shower.
- Gardening and simplifying your life will reduce pitta ailments.

## HERB: *Tendonitis Ointment*

Chickweed is actually a powerful anti-inflammatory agent that works well on arthritic-type disabilities. Chickweed has antirheumatic properties that make it the go-to herb for tendonitis. It also grows right in your backyard!

½ CUP CHICKWEED

1 CUP OLIVE OIL

1–2 OUNCES BEESWAX

½ TEASPOON VITAMIN E OIL

Pack the herbs into the olive oil and cook on low on the stovetop for one and a half hours. Strain through cheesecloth into a glass bowl and add one ounce of beeswax. Stir until beeswax is melted, then add vitamin E and stir again. Pour a drop of the mixture onto the counter. Run your finger through the drop after a few seconds of cooling: if it is too thick, add a little oil; if it is too thin, add a little more beeswax. Once you are happy with the consistency, pour into a jar and label. Cool before applying to skin. Apply to desired area by rubbing or massaging into the skin. You may cover with gauze if desired to protect furniture and clothing. Repeat application morning and night. Store in containers with tight-fitting lids in a cool, dark area for up to one year.

## ESSENTIAL OIL: *Tendonitis Roll-On*

Tendonitis pain levels often reach a level eight or more on the pain score. These oils work well at reducing pain with their analgesic and anti-inflammatory properties. This recipe is strong, so do a patch test first and ensure with your physician that these essential oils won't interfere with your current medications.

10 DROPS WINTERGREEN OIL

10 DROPS BIRCH OIL

5 DROPS HELICHRYSUM

5 DROPS PEPPERMINT

1 OUNCE CARRIER OIL (SUCH AS JOJOBA, SESAME, GRAPESEED, OR YOUR PREFERENCE)

4 DROPS VITAMIN E OIL

Mix all of the ingredients in a small container. Place the ingredients into a roll-on bottle and label it. Shake well before each usage. Roll around the painful area. You may cover with gauze or a bandage to protect furniture and clothing. Repeat as pain returns. Do not apply to mucus membranes, open wounds, genitals, or other sensitive areas. Store in a cool, dark area for up to six months.

## HOME REMEDY: *Tendonitis Vinegar Wrap*

Vinegar is a great anti-inflammatory agent to apply to tendonitis, especially in the elbows and knees. This wrap has been used for ages to reduce the swelling and pain of tendonitis.

**½ CUP WATER**

**½ CUP APPLE CIDER VINEGAR**

**LONG PIECE OF MUSLIN OR COTTON**

Combine the ingredients in a medium-sized bowl. Stir well. Apply the mixture to a long piece of muslin or cotton. Wrap the treated material around the wrist, knee, ankle, etc., and leave for at least fifteen minutes or until temperature is uncomfortable. Reapply as needed.

• • • •

# THYROID

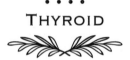

The thyroid is a small gland in your neck that controls the thyroid hormone. The thyroid gland controls your metabolism, heartbeat, etc. Fatigue, weight gain, weight loss, and confusion are all symptoms of a thyroid disorder. Getting your thyroid regulated is optimal to good health. Through the centuries, home remedies, essential oils, herbs, and Ayurveda have been used worldwide to control the thyroid gland and get it back to optimal peak performance.

## AYURVEDA: *Meditation*

Thyroid imbalance can cause emotional turmoil. Meditation and yoga can help you keep calm, centered, and grounded when going through the worst of times. Try this meditation practice to bring your hormones and mood back to normal.

Find a room or a place outdoors that is free of all distractions. Make it a place you feel calm and comfortable in. Play a soothing type of music if you desire. Sit on the floor, on a pillow or a rug. Cross your legs and place your hands, palms up, on your knees.

Close your eyes. Banish negative thoughts and replace them with positive, peaceful thoughts. This is a cycle you may have to repeat a hundred times to get out the "bad" and bring in the "good." Every time a negative thought enters your mind, just push it aside.

Concentrate on your breathing. Take long, slow breaths in through your nose, hold the breath in your lungs for a few seconds, and then release with longer slower breaths through your mouth.

Repeat this process for about ten minutes. Stress, anxiety, and worry will fade away, and strength, happiness, and well-being will take its place.

## HERB: *The Thyroid Regulator*

These herbs contain natural hormone-balancing properties to help you recover some of those lost hormones due to a thyroid disorder. This decoction is easy to make and very effective for many people.

> 1 TEASPOON ECHINACEA ROOT
>
> 1 TEASPOON BLADDERWRACK
>
> 1 TEASPOON LEMON BALM
>
> 1 PINT BOILING WATER
>
> HONEY (OPTIONAL)

Place the herbs into a mason jar. Pour one pint of boiling water over the herbs. Allow herbs to steep, covered, for twenty minutes or more. Strain the mixture and discard the herbs. Add honey, if desired. Drink the mixture slowly over the course of a few hours. Repeat daily until desired results are achieved. Remainder may be kept in a jar with a tight-fitting lid in the refrigerator for up to three days.

## ESSENTIAL OIL: *Thyroid Rub*

These oils have worked for many people in getting the thyroid functioning properly again. Use this rub daily and notice if your weight fluctuations are controlled and if your sluggishness disappears.

8 DROPS LEMON BALM (MELISSA) OIL

8 DROPS LIME OIL

8 DROPS GRAPEFRUIT OIL

8 DROPS GERANIUM OIL

5 DROPS VITAMIN E OIL

½ OUNCE CARRIER OIL (SUCH AS JOJOBA, SESAME, GRAPESEED, OR YOUR PREFERENCE)

Mix the ingredients in a small glass container and apply lightly to the area desired, such as pressure points, neck, soles of feet, temples, and chest. Keep essential oil mixture away from open wounds, mucus membranes, genitals, eyes, and sensitive areas. Repeat application as needed, usually two to three times daily. Store unused portion in a glass jar with a tight-fitting lid, label it, and keep it in a cool, dark area for up to six months.

### HOME REMEDY: *Thyroid Balance*

Thyroid disorder affects mostly women. For hundreds of years, women have developed ways to create hormone balance to the thyroid gland. These tips and hints are tried and true healing methods for thyroid disorder:

- Take vitamins A and B.
- Eat peanuts, eggs, carrots, green veggies, and fat.
- Do not eat gas-producing veggies or cruciferous vegetables such as cauliflower, broccoli, radishes, beans, and soy.
- Low carb diets work wonders on thyroid disorder.
- Eat ginger, coconut oil, ghee, avocadoes, and apple cider vinegar as often as possible.
- Meditate, pray, and exercise.
- Get out in nature. Go for a walk. Garden. Play with the children outside. Vitamin D is abundant through the sun and can help to regulate hormones.

• • • •

# TINNITUS

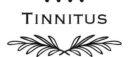

Tinnitus is annoying and can interfere in all areas of your life. The cause can stem from various diseases to hearing loss, so getting a diagnosis from your doctor can sometimes lead to solutions for healing. Making that horrible ringing stop can often be easily remedied with one of these simple recipes.

## AYURVEDA: *Tinnitus Pull*

In Ayurveda it is believed that tinnitus is caused by an overabundance of toxins in the body, and in the head, teeth, and mouth in particular. This oil-pulling remedy takes the toxins and adheres them to the oil. Spitting out the oil also removes the toxins from the mouth, thereby easing tinnitus symptoms. Sunflower seed oil also provides additional benefits of vitamins A and E.

### 1 TEASPOON SUNFLOWER SEED OIL

Place the spoonful of oil in your mouth and very gently swish oil between all teeth, over tongue, and in all areas of the mouth for ten to fifteen minutes. After you are done, spit all of the oil out of your mouth and into the garbage. Do not swallow oil. Repeat every morning as needed.

## HERB: *Daily Tinnitus Infusion*

These two herbs have been reported to stop tinnitus in many people easily and effectively. This infusion is pleasant to taste, so it is not a chore to drink it. The healing properties in this recipe promote all-around good health.

### 2 CUPS WATER

### ¼ CUP CALENDULA FLOWERS

### ¼ CUP PLANTAIN

Bring water to a boil. Place herbs in a mason jar and pour the boiling water over them, cover, and leave eight to ten hours or overnight. Strain and, if desired, add sweetener of choice. Compost or discard herbs. Drink one or two cups daily. Store remainder in the refrigerator, in a jar with a tight-fitting lid, for up to two days.

## ESSENTIAL OIL: *Tinnitus Massage*

Tinnitus is often associated with stress. This balm has sedative and tranquilizing properties and relaxes the entire body. This massage is reported to relieve tinnitus while giving you a good night's sleep at the same time.

**7 DROPS LEMON BALM (MELISSA) OIL**

**7 DROPS ROSEMARY OIL**

**½ OUNCE CARRIER OIL (SUCH AS JOJOBA, SESAME, GRAPESEED, OR YOUR PREFERENCE)**

**4 DROPS VITAMIN E OIL**

Mix the ingredients in a small glass container and apply lightly to the outer ear and neck areas. Using an old pillowcase is recommended in order to protect your linen. Keep essential oil mixture away from inner ear canal, open wounds, mucus membranes, genitals, eyes, and sensitive areas. Repeat application as needed, usually two to three times daily. Store unused portion in a glass jar with a tight-fitting lid, label it, and keep it in a cool, dark area for up to six months.

## HOME REMEDY: *Tinnitus Shot*

This home remedy is very old but has been known to have a good effect on tinnitus. It does not taste pleasant to most people, but sometimes it's worth it to make that ringing stop. Try drinking this shot every morning for a while and notice if your spells of tinnitus decrease or stop altogether.

**1 TABLESPOON WATER**

**1 TABLESPOON APPLE CIDER VINEGAR**

**1 TEASPOON HONEY (OPTIONAL)**

Mix the ingredients together into a very small glass or a shot glass and drink rapidly, all at once.

. . . .
# TONSILLITIS (AND ADENOIDS)

Children often have sore throats, and the adenoids and tonsils are oftentimes the culprit. Adenoids and tonsils are usually removed at the same time if repeated infections occur. These masses of tissues can swell, become inflamed and infected, and cause tremendous pain along with labored breathing. Inflammation can occur for many reasons such as viruses, bacteria, sinus infections, and even the common cold. There are many remedies available to ease the pain, aid in sleep, and reduce the inflammation. Use caution and seek medical attention if fever, chills, or severe pain are present.

## AYURVEDA: *Ayurvedic Salty Gargle*

In Ayurveda natural ingredients are the best ingredients. The salt of the earth is one of the most natural and healing medicines known. This remedy heals all sorts of throat conditions.

### 1 TEASPOON SEA SALT OR SALT OF CHOICE

### ¼ CUP LUKEWARM WATER

Slowly stir the salt into the water until it has dissolved. Put a small amount into your mouth and rapidly swish around and gargle in the back of the throat as much as possible without swallowing. Spit it all out when done. Repeat throughout the day as pain returns. Discard any remainder at the end of the day.

## HERB: *Tonsil Herbal Tea*

When adenoids and tonsils are swollen, swallowing and breathing can become difficult. This remedy has herbs that contain antibiotic, antiseptic, antibacterial, and anti-inflammatory properties as well as immunity-boosting agents. The warm tea is also soothing as it goes down.

### 1 CUP WATER

### 1 TEASPOON SAGE LEAVES

### 1 TEASPOON ECHINACEA FLOWERS

Bring water to a boil, then add herbs. Remove from heat, cover, and steep for six to eight minutes. Strain and, if desired, add sweetener of choice. Compost or discard herbs.

## ESSENTIAL OIL: *Healing Oil Throat Rub*

This recipe brings so much relief and comfort to someone in pain. The healing components of this blend contain analgesic, anesthetic, anti-infectious, anti-inflammatory, antiseptic, and febrifuge properties.

- 3 DROPS SAGE OIL
- 3 DROPS PEPPERMINT OIL
- 3 DROPS GARLIC OIL
- 1 OUNCE CARRIER OIL (SUCH AS JOJOBA, SESAME, GRAPESEED, OR YOUR PREFERENCE)
- 4 DROPS VITAMIN E OIL

Mix the ingredients in a small glass container and apply lightly to the area desired, such as throat, soles of feet, temples, and chest. Keep essential oil mixture away from open wounds, mucus membranes, genitals, eyes, and sensitive areas. Repeat application as needed, usually two to three times daily. Store unused portion in a glass jar with a tight-fitting lid, label it, and keep it in a cool, dark area for up to six months.

## HOME REMEDY: *Tonsillitis Remedy*

When I was young, my grandmother used teas and spoons to dish out the medications that she made in her kitchen. Usually we felt better immediately just knowing that she was mixing up something special and magical just for us. This old-time remedy works wonders, and the honey gives it an added boost of flavor. These ingredients contain powerful antibacterial, anti-inflammatory, and analgesic properties to help with reducing the pain, swelling, and infection of the adenoids and tonsils.

- 1 GARLIC CLOVE, PULVERIZED
- 1 TEASPOON HONEY
- 5 DROPS LEMON JUICE

Mash all of the ingredients together in a large spoon. Take a spoonful by mouth and repeat process twice daily until no more pain or infection is present. If pain or fever persists, seek medical attention.

• • • •

## TOOTHACHE

When swelling and infection are present, a dentist must perform treatments to stop the infection. Dental pain can be excruciating. If you can't get to your dentist as soon as you'd like, then try one of these essential oil, home remedy, herbal, or Ayurvedic treatments.

### AYURVEDA: *Tooth Swab*

This old remedy has been used forever in ending the pain of toothache until you can get to a dentist. It doesn't taste good, but when you are in that much pain, taste is sometimes irrelevant. This clove recipe is easy to make and has all of the anti-inflammatory, analgesic, and healing properties of clove essential oil, but you make the oils yourself.

**5 CLOVE BUDS**

**1 TABLESPOON COCONUT OIL**

Grind the cloves as well as possible and add to coconut oil. Stir constantly over low heat and simmer for five minutes. Remove from heat and strain the oil through cheesecloth. Discard the cloves, retaining the oil. Dip a cotton swab into the cooled oil and apply to toothache. Try to keep tongue away from tooth after application. Repeat as needed until dental treatment is obtained.

### HERB: *Flower Pain Killer*

Lavender and chamomile are known for their beauty, aroma, and sleep-inducing charms, but they are also powerful painkillers. Try this tea when you have a toothache to eliminate pain and invite peace and calm. It's best to drink this tea at bedtime or when you have some down time. Don't drive or operated machinery when drinking this relaxing tea.

**1 CUP WATER**

**½ TEASPOON CHAMOMILE FLOWERS**

**½ TEASPOON LAVENDER FLOWERS**

Bring water to a boil, then add herbs. Remove from heat, cover, and steep for six to eight minutes. Strain and, if desired, add sweetener of choice. Compost or discard herbs.

## ESSENTIAL OIL: *Toothache Oil*

Clove has been a toothache cure-all for thousands of years. Clove has anti-inflammatory, analgesic, and healing compounds to help stop the pain in its tracks until you can get to the dentist. Ensure that your clove oils are 100 percent therapeutic and safe for internal usage.

**2 DROPS CLOVE OIL**

**1 PIECE GAUZE**

Drip the clove oil onto the gauze. Fold the gauze and hold it between the teeth that are inflamed. Try not to let it touch your tongue, as clove burns and tastes horrible. Discard after using for an hour. Repeat as needed.

## HOME REMEDY: *Ginger Tooth Compress*

This is probably the easiest recipe in the entire universe. Ginger is loaded with anti-inflammatory and anti-infective properties. Placing it straight on the tooth allows all of these healing properties to be absorbed through the gums and into the inflamed areas needed.

**½-INCH GINGER ROOT**

Peel the ginger root. Take the very tender flesh inside and grind a very small amount. Roll into a tiny ball and place ginger on tooth or hold it between top and bottom teeth over painful area. Hold in place for ten to twenty minutes, then spit it out. The remainder of the ginger can be placed into an airtight bag and refrigerated up to one week.

• • • •
# ULCERS (MOUTH)

Mouth ulcers are red or white swollen areas of the inner cheeks and gums that are painful and seem to last forever. Any number of things can cause a mouth ulcer: heredity, celiac disease, dental wounds, bacteria, cuts, toothpaste, or allergies. These painful ulcers are not serious unless they become infected, in which case a trip to the doctor's office may be in order.

### AYURVEDA: *Tomato Ulcer Cure*

Tomatoes contain acids that fight inflammation and promote healing. This Ayurvedic cure for mouth ulcers can be as tasty as it is healing.

**1 LARGE TOMATO**

**¼ CUP WATER**

Peel and core the tomato. Place the tomato and the water into a blender and blend until smooth. Take one tablespoon at a time and swish around in mouth, making sure to coat the ulcer with the liquid several times. Spit out juice when done. Repeat this process at least three times daily until ulcer heals. Store remainder in a jar with a tight-fitting lid, in the refrigerator, for up to forty-eight hours.

### HERB: *Make-Ahead Ulcer Tincture*

This ancient tincture recipe uses dandelion's healing properties to treat mouth ulcers and bring about rapid relief.

**½ CUP DANDELION STEMS AND LEAVES**

**1 PINT VODKA OR VEGETABLE GLYCERIN**

Place herbs in a pint jar until it's half full with dried herbs or two-thirds full with fresh herbs, and cover the herbs with a high proof vodka (for adults) or vegetable glycerin (for children), leaving about an inch at the top of the jar. Cover tightly and place in a cool, dark location. Shake vigorously every day for two weeks, then let it set without shaking for one month. Strain, bottle, label, and put the date you decanted it, or strained out the herb. Drink a half to one dropperful in tea, water, juice, or other liquid two to three times daily until ulcer is cleared. If kept in a cool, dark place, tincture made with alcohol will last several years and vegetable glycerin-based tincture will last up to one year.

## ESSENTIAL OIL: *Tea Tree Gargle*

Tea tree is loaded with antibacterial, antiviral, vulnerary, and anti-inflammatory agents to treat mouth ulcers. Ensure that your tea tree oil is 100 percent therapeutic grade and labeled as okay for internal usage.

**4 DROPS TEA TREE OIL**

**1 TABLESPOON WATER**

Combine ingredients into a glass. Put a small amount into your mouth and rapidly swish around, taking special care to swish over the ulcer several times. Spit it all out when done. Do not swallow. Store remainder in a jar with a tight-fitting lid, in a cool, dark area, for up to twenty-four hours.

## HOME REMEDY: *Ulcer Begone Tips*

Home remedies abound to rid oneself of mouth ulcers. Everyone in my family had a different opinion and sworn testimonies about how they had previously ridded themselves of mouth ulcers. Here are a few of their tips that did prove to have ulcer-healing benefits:

- Place a pinch of alum on the ulcer and let it remain. Repeat twice daily until ulcer is gone.
- Take extra vitamins E, A, and B12.
- Drink cold milk and let it sit in the mouth, covering the ulcer.
- Grind bananas or cabbage and let the food rest on ulcer before swallowing.
- Take a few drops of honey and place on the ulcer. Repeat every time you think of it, all day long.
- Grind up a basil leaf, apply it to the ulcer, and leave on for at least ten minutes. Repeat twice daily.

. . . .

# VAGINAL ITCH

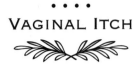

Vaginal itch can be uncomfortable, painful, and embarrassing. Women have healed themselves of vaginal itch throughout the centuries with a wide variety of healing methods. Vaginal itch can be caused by anything from food allergies to hygiene. Try one of these remedies the next time you experience vaginal itch to bring some instant relief to your nether regions.

### AYURVEDA: *Itch Recipe*

This is the simplest, easiest cure ever! Coconut oil has numerous healing and relieving properties.

Apply a half teaspoon coconut oil to the outer vaginal area that is itchy. Lie on a towel and allow to air-dry. Ensure through locked doors that you won't be interrupted in this calming position. After thirty minutes rinse with tepid water and thoroughly pat dry.

### HERB: *Rosemary Wash*

This recipe is exactly as it is titled: a cleansing, healing, cooling wash with the itch-eradicating power of rosemary. This wash is best performed when you first notice the itching.

**3 TABLESPOONS ROSEMARY NEEDLES**

**2 CUPS BOILING WATER**

Place the herbs into the boiling water. Remove from heat, cover, and steep for twenty to thirty minutes. Strain liquid into a large bowl. Discard herbs. Add ice cubes to water if it is not cool enough. Soak a soft piece of linen or material in the liquid and wring it out lightly. Placing yourself on a towel or in the shower, gently wash the vaginal area with the liquid. Do not rub hard, as it could tear delicate skin. Allow to air-dry. Repeat as needed all day. Discard any remainder.

## ESSENTIAL OIL: *Salty Oil Soak*

The healing properties of these oils can bring rapid relief. The salt is healing and vulnerary as well. The next time you have vaginal itch that drives you crazy, soak in this tub and come out cool, clean, and confidant.

> **3 CUPS SALTS (PINK HIMALAYAN, SEA, EPSOM, OR YOUR PREFERENCE)**
>
> **10 DROPS LAVENDER OIL**
>
> **10 DROPS TEA TREE OIL**
>
> **5 DROPS BERGAMOT OIL**
>
> **1 TABLESPOON CARRIER OIL (SUCH AS JOJOBA, SESAME, GRAPESEED, OR YOUR PREFERENCE)**
>
> **1 TABLESPOON MILK (OPTIONAL)**

Combine salts and oils, stirring until well blended. Cover tightly. Leave mixture in a dark area for twenty-four hours, then stir again. Run the bath-water, but not too hot as to ruin the oils. Add a half cup of the bath salt mixture to bathwater. If you add milk to the water, it will prevent the oil from floating on top of the water and sticking to your skin. Store unused portion in a glass jar with a tight-fitting lid, label it, and keep it in a cool, dark area for up to three months.

## HOME REMEDY: *Itchin' and Witchin'*

Some of these cures worked so well in the Middle Ages that women who shared their recipes were thought to be witches! No magic is required, however; there are actually healing properties and common sense associated with each of these remedies.

- Do not scratch the itch. It will only make it spread and become infected.
- Wear loose clothing that allows the air to circulate.
- Wear white cotton panties.
- Take a bath with a cup of apple cider vinegar added to it.
- Avoid chemicals.
- Eat yogurt every day.

- Do not eat any sugar. Sugar breeds yeast, which in turn can cause vaginal itching.

- Check for food allergies. Try the elimination diet to ensure you are not allergic to the main culprits of wheat, dairy, or red meat.

• • • •
## VERTIGO

There are many reasons why a person can suffer from vertigo. That dizzy, nauseous feeling that can hit you from out of the blue is more common than you may think. Essential oils, herbs, home remedies, and Ayurveda have all been used for thousands of years to reduce vertigo's effects.

### AYURVEDA: *Tree Pose for Balance*

In Ayurveda it is believed that focusing and strengthening one's balance will give you control over vertigo spells. When you don't have vertigo, try this tree pose every day. When you do have a spell of vertigo, attempt to do the pose and it will help you to regain your balance and focus.

Stand in a comfortable area, with your feet flat on the floor. Bring your hands to your chest in prayer position, with your elbows out to the side.

Close your eyes or focus on an object in front of you.

Take even, steady breaths in and out throughout this pose.

Slowly bring one foot up and rest it on the calf of the opposite leg for a count of three breaths. Ensure that your foot does not rest on your knee, but on your calf. Once you have balance, you may raise your hands over your head and focus on slow, steady breathing. Repeat entire sequence two times on each side.

When you have learned to balance and focus from this exercise, challenge yourself with bringing your foot up to the opposite thigh instead of the calf, and complete the pose in that position.

## HERB: *Vertigo Tincture*

This tincture has tons of anti-inflammatory and antinausea elements to help keep vertigo under control. It's simple to make and very healing for all aspects of your health.

**10–15 GARLIC CLOVES, PEELED AND ROUGHLY CHOPPED**

**3 LARGE GINGER ROOTS, ROUGHLY CHOPPED**

**1 PINT VODKA OR VEGETABLE GLYCERIN**

Place herbs in a pint jar until it's half full with dried herbs or two-thirds full with fresh herbs, and cover the herbs with a high proof vodka (for adults) or vegetable glycerin (for children), leaving about an inch at the top of the jar. Cover tightly and place in a cool, dark location. Shake vigorously every day for two weeks, then let it set without shaking for one month. Strain, bottle, label, and put the date you decanted it, or strained out the herb. Drink a half to one dropperful in tea, water, juice, or other liquid two to three times daily until vertigo is cleared. If kept in a cool, dark place, tincture made with alcohol will last several years and vegetable glycerin-based tincture will last up to one year.

## ESSENTIAL OIL: *Vertigo Inhale*

Many people have had great success keeping vertigo under control simply by inhaling some peppermint. Carry a small vial in your purse, car, or office, and the next time that dizziness hits, just uncork and smell. You can also apply a drop of oil to the palm of your hand, an oil inhaler, or a tissue. Bring close to your nostrils and inhale the aroma deeply. This process sends the properties straight to your brain and the effects are immediate. You can complete this procedure three or four times daily.

## HOME REMEDY: *Vertigo Salad*

The ingredients in this salad have long been thought to stave off bouts of vertigo as well as help diminish the dizziness and nausea that accompany it.

**1 CUP DARK LEAFY GREEN LETTUCE**

**5 BASIL LEAVES**

**4 STRAWBERRIES, SLICED**

1 GARLIC CLOVE, MINCED

JUICE OF 1 LEMON

½ TEASPOON HONEY

Chop the lettuce and the basil leaves and add to a salad bowl. Place the sliced strawberries on top. Finely mince the garlic clove and add to the lemon juice and honey. Whisk remaining ingredients into a dressing. Pour over the salad. Store any remainder in the refrigerator for up to twenty-four hours.

• • • •

# VIRUS

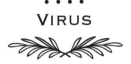

A virus is usually an infection of the lungs, throat, or stomach that is passed from person to person through airborne germs. Essential oils, Ayurveda, home remedies, and herbs can help, not only with the pain, nausea, and discomfort of a viral infection, but they can actually protect a person's surroundings so that the virus cannot survive to be passed on to anyone else. Viral infections are very contagious, and it seems entire towns can become infected. A good way to protect your family is to begin using these treatments in the home once you know flu and virus season has begun.

## AYURVEDA: *Virus Milk*

This recipe can heal and protect you and your surroundings from viral airborne germs. It is full of antimicrobial, antibacterial, and anti-inflammatory properties. Drink this, then rest while the healing properties work to banish those horrible little virus germs.

1 CUP MILK

1 TEASPOON TURMERIC

1 PINCH BLACK PEPPER

Warm the milk slightly on the stove or in the microwave. Stir in the turmeric and black pepper. When cool enough, drink warm milk mixture. Discard any remainder. Repeat as needed.

## HERB: *Virus Blocker*

This decoction helps to control dizziness and nausea and has been used by hundreds of cultures since people first began experiencing viral infections. Nettle has antiviral properties to give you that boost you need. Try making up a batch of this recipe to drink slowly throughout the day to prevent or heal a virus.

½ CUP NETTLE LEAVES

1 CUP BOILING WATER

HONEY (OPTIONAL)

Place the herbs into a mason jar. Pour 1 cup of boiling water over the herbs. Allow herbs to steep in water for twenty minutes or more. Strain the mixture and discard the herbs. Add honey, if desired. Drink the decoction slowly over the course of a few hours. Repeat twice daily until desired results are achieved. Remainder may be kept in a jar with a tight-fitting lid in the refrigerator for up to three days.

## ESSENTIAL OIL: *Spray Protector*

These essential oils contain analgesic, antifungal, anti-infective, antimicrobial, antiviral, and anti-inflammatory properties. This spray will protect you from the virus germs or help banish it once you are already infected. You can spray this almost everywhere. Shake well before each use to combine the ingredients.

10 DROPS TEA TREE OIL

10 DROPS EUCALYPTUS OIL

5 DROPS MARJORAM OIL

5 DROPS CLOVE OIL

5 DROPS ORANGE OIL

1 TABLESPOON WITCH HAZEL

4 OUNCES WATER

Add all ingredients to a dark-colored spray bottle to prevent sunlight from damaging contents. Shake bottle and spray onto area desired, such as body, hair, home, car, or office. Do not spray into open wounds, genitals, eyes, or mucus membranes. Store in a cool, dark area for up to three months.

## HOME REMEDY: *Common-Sense Virus Tips*

These are some common-sense tips used around the world to prevent or treat viruses. Try incorporating a few of these during virus and flu season.

- Stay hydrated.

- Rest often, as needed.

- Make sure you get 7–8 hours of sleep a night.

- Take time to meditate and pray.

- De-stress however you are able: walk in nature, do yoga, read a book.

- Wash your hands often and well.

- Avoid public restrooms when possible.

- Eat fresh fruit and vegetables daily.

- Never share combs, brushes, hats, or clothing with others.

- Always take exercise in one form or another each and every day.

- Always cover your mouth when you cough, and try to cough into the crook of your elbow.

- Wipe down phones, counters, and door knobs weekly with a wash combining essential oils and water such as Spray Protector on page 286.

· · · · ·

# WARTS

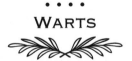

Warts can be caused by viruses, heredity, or sometimes for no discernable reason at all. People have tried ridding themselves of warts for ages and are often successful at their own endeavors. Here are a few of the ways that various cultures put an end to those ugly patches of malformed skin.

## AYURVEDA: *Springtime Wart Killer*

This old Ayurvedic recipe works very well, but only in the springtime when dandelions pepper your yard. Pick a dandelion from your yard. Run your finger and thumb from the flower end of the stem all the way to the bottom, catching the sap that flows from the tube-like stem. Apply the sap to the wart and cover with a bandage. Allow to remain on until next application. Reapply sap twice daily for two weeks.

## HERB: *Wart Remedy*

This old herbal remedy works quickly and effectively at shriveling up a wart and causing it to die. This recipe has been used in numerous cultures many times with success. It's easy and you have everything you need already in your kitchen. Warts cannot survive in this blend and will die.

**3 GARLIC CLOVES, MACERATED**

**1 OUNCE APPLE CIDER VINEGAR**

One the stovetop, heat the garlic and apple cider vinegar on low for up to ten minutes. Remove from heat and allow to cool. Wash wart area with mixture. Allow to air-dry. Repeat process three to five times daily for two weeks. Store remainder in refrigerator for up to one week.

## ESSENTIAL OIL: *Anti-Wart Blend*

This is the essential oil recipe I used to successfully rid myself of a small wart that formed next to a wart I had gotten removed in the doctor's office (yes, warts can come back).

**10 DROPS TEA TREE OIL**

**10 DROPS LEMON OIL**

**½ OUNCE CARRIER OIL (SUCH AS JOJOBA, SESAME, GRAPESEED, OR YOUR PREFERENCE)**

**5 DROPS VITAMIN E OIL**

Mix the ingredients in a small glass container and apply lightly to the wart. Cover with a bandage. Keep essential oil mixture away from open wounds, mucus membranes, genitals, eyes, and sensitive areas. Repeat application as needed, usually two to three times daily. Store unused portion in a glass jar with a tight-fitting lid, label it, and keep it in a cool, dark area for up to six months.

## HOME REMEDY: *Wart Home Remedy*

The secret behind this home remedy is that warts are said to be living, breathing viruses. Once you cut off the air supply, the wart is said to dry up and die.

This remedy might be a little painful, but old-timers swear by it. Place a piece of duct tape on the wart. Rub the area often to flatten and smooth the tape to the wart. After seven to ten days, slowly peel off tape. A scabby, dried-up wart will remain and can be removed as pieces flake off.

• • • •

# WOUNDS (CUTS AND BLEEDING)

There are as many ways to get small wounds as there are recipes to heal them. Bumping your leg, the slip of a knife, falling and hurting yourself are all ways to end up with a little burn, cut, or bruise. Small wounds can be treated at home, but major wounds with excessive blood loss or infection should be treated at the ER. These are my favorite wound recipes from around the world and have worked wonders on my family. Most of these recipes have only one or two ingredients. They are simple but work so well at healing and preventing infections.

## AYURVEDA: *Coconut Wound Healer*

In Ayurveda the best ingredients are the simplest ingredients. Coconut oil has cicatrisant and healing properties. Use this the next time you have a minor wound to speed up healing.

½ TEASPOON COCONUT OIL

1 PIECE GAUZE OR BANDAGE

Apply a thin layer of coconut oil directly to the minor cut. Layer a piece of gauze or bandage over the area to avoid staining clothing or furniture with the oil. Leave on for several hours and reapply as needed.

## HERB: *Herbal Wound Wash*

This soothing, cooling wash keeps the area germ-free, prevents infections, stops bleeding and pain, and also smells good. These herbs have astringent, anti-inflammatory, vulnerary, and vasodilator properties to stop bleeding and fight against infections.

> 1 CUP WATER
>
> 1½ TABLESPOONS CALENDULA FLOWERS
>
> 1½ TABLESPOONS RASPBERRY LEAF
>
> 1 TABLESPOON WITCH HAZEL

Bring water to a boil, then add herbs. Reduce heat to low and simmer for twenty minutes. Remove from heat and strain. Discard herbs and cool liquid to room temperature. Add witch hazel to mixture. Use the liquid as a wash for the affected area. Reapply as often as needed. Store remainder in refrigerator for up to twenty-four hours in a jar or bowl with a tight-fitting lid.

## ESSENTIAL OIL: *Styptic Oil Salve*

The essential oils used here have hemostatic, cicatrisant, vulnerary, anti-infective, and anti-inflammatory healing properties.

> 5 DROPS YARROW OIL
>
> 5 DROPS GERANIUM OIL
>
> 3 DROPS VITAMIN E OIL
>
> ½ OUNCE CARRIER OIL (SUCH AS JOJOBA, SESAME, GRAPESEED, OR YOUR PREFERENCE)

Mix the ingredients in a small glass container and apply lightly to the wound area. Cover wound with bandage. Keep essential oil mixture away from large open or deep wounds, mucus membranes, genitals, eyes, and sensitive areas. Repeat application as needed, usually two to three times daily. Store unused portion in a glass jar with a tight-fitting lid, label it, and keep it in a cool, dark area for up to six months.

## HOME REMEDY: *Homemade Bandage Salve*

Not only is yarrow beautiful to look at, but it provides about as much anti-inflammatory and anti-infective properties as any other plant or chemical on earth. I usually make a few jars of this healing blend every summer, and by the next year I need it again. We put it on everything from bruises, wounds, and sprains to arthritis, cuts, and insect stings!

1 CUP CARRIER OIL (SUCH AS JOJOBA, SESAME, GRAPESEED, OR YOUR PREFERENCE)

½ CUP YARROW LEAVES

10 DROPS VITAMIN E OIL

Preheat oven to 225 degrees. Put the carrier oil in an oven-safe dish. Stir in the herbs. Place the dish in the oven, shut the door, and turn off the oven. Leave the oil in the oven for three to four hours. Cool completely. Strain through cheesecloth, discard herbs into compost pile, and add the vitamin E oil. Bottle and label. Apply a few drops to bandage or gauze and place securely onto wound for up to eight hours. Repeat as needed. Store in a cool, dark area in a jar with a tight-fitting lid for up to one year.

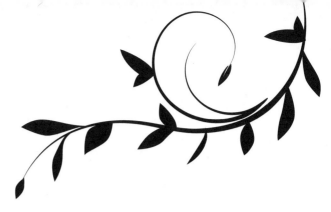

# CONCLUSION

Writing *Llewellyn's Book of Natural Remedies* has been a great experience for me. I hope you have gained some knowledge about how to use natural healing to benefit you and your loved ones in times of need. Knowledge about natural healing is a very powerful tool for you to have. Keep building on what you have learned and become that source of information that people can turn to when they feel they have nowhere else to go.

Learning to use common sense, a few kitchen ingredients, and willpower, you can overcome some of the most common ailments that plague humans. Learning from other cultures, beliefs, and time spans, we can often conquer something that big pharma can't. I urge you to experiment and adapt natural healing methods to your own life. Taking control of your health can be very beneficial.

As time progresses and we leave more and more of our healthcare decisions up to insurance providers and pharmaceutical companies, we lose what we have been born with: the will to live naturally, without chemicals, and the ability to make our own healthcare decisions. We can use our brains and our knowledge to combat disease in a healthier, more natural, and non-invasive way. I do believe in integrative medicine for serious health issues, but I also believe that we rely on "the system" way too much for our everyday ailments.

*Llewellyn's Book of Natural Remedies* is meant as a tool for you to gain insightful knowledge about yourself and the world around you. Practice what you have learned, and you and yours can look forward to a future that is stronger and healthier and has less intervention from outsiders who do not truly know you. Know yourself and learn.

Much healing to you,
*Vannoy*

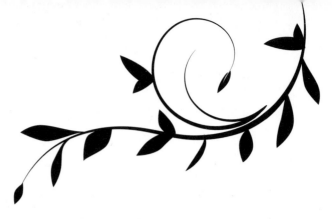

# GLOSSARY

**ANALGESIC:** lowers pain

**APERIENT:** relieves constipation

**ANTIALLERGENIC:** assists in lowering allergy symptoms

**ANTIBACTERIAL:** destroys bacteria and reduces the ability of bacteria to reproduce

**ANTIBIOTIC:** assists in fighting bacterial infections

**ANTICARCINOGENIC:** contains cancer-fighting properties

**ANTICATARRHAL:** removes excess mucus in the body and assists with respiratory ailments

**ANTIDEPRESSANT:** assists in alleviating depression

**ANTIEMETIC:** soothes upset stomach and relieves nausea and vomiting

**ANTIFUNGAL:** assists in relieving the itching and spreading of fungal attacks

**ANTI-INFECTIVE:** fights infection

**ANTI-INFLAMMATORY:** cools and relieves inflamed areas

**ANTI-IRRITANT:** reduces inflammatory or irritating skin

**ANTIMICROBIAL:** inhibits the growth of microorganisms

**ANTIOXIDANT:** reduces oxidation or deterioration of products

**ANTIPARASITIC:** treats parasitic diseases

**ANTIPHLOGISTIC:** reduces inflammation

**ANTIRHEUMATIC:** reduces arthritis pain and swelling

**ANTISEBORRHEIC:** relieves dandruff or dry skin

**ANTISEPTIC:** assists in fighting germs and infections

**ANTISPASMODIC:** relieves spasms and cramping

**ANTITUMOR:** contains tumer-relieving agents

**ANTITUSSIVE:** relieves coughs and respiratory ailments

**ANTIVENOUS:** prevents blood clots

**ANTIVIRAL:** used to treat viral infections

**APHRODISIAC:** increases sexual desire

**ASTRINGENT:** contracts and tightens tissues

**AROMATIC:** imparts a pleasing aroma

**BACTERICIDAL:** kills living bacteria

**BALSAMIC:** contains balsam oil

**BECHIC:** relieves coughs

**CARMINATIVE:** relieves bloating and gas

**CEPHALIC:** relates to head injuries and illness

**CHOLAGOGUE:** promotes discharge and flow of bile

**CICATRISANT:** good for cell regeneration, heals scars

**CIRCULATORY STIMULANT:** promotes better blood circulation

**CORDIAL:** warm and comforting

**CYTOPHYLACTIC:** stimulates new skin cells; beneficial for aging and mature skin

**DECONGESTANT:** reduces nasal mucus production and swelling

**DETOXIFYING:** removes toxins from the body

**DIAPHORETIC:** induces perspiration

**DIURETIC:** promotes discharge of urine and rids the body of water

**EMOLLIENT:** softens and smooths the skin

**EXPECTORANT:** removes excess mucus from the respiratory system

**EMMENAGOGUE:** induces menstruation

**FEBRIFUGE:** reduces fever

**FUNGICIDAL:** inhibits the growth of fungus

**GALACTAGOGUE:** promotes lactation

**HEPATIC:** beneficial to liver

**HEMOSTATIC:** stops the flow of blood

**HYPERTENSIVE:** lowers blood pressure

**HYPOTENSIVE:** raises blood pressure

**LYMPHATIC:** relates to lymph secretions

**MUCOLYTIC:** sedative and helps to break down mucus

**NERVINE:** calms and soothes nervous system

**OPTHALMIC:** beneficial for eyes

**PARTURIENT:** refers to a woman in labor

**RUBEFACIENT:** causes skin to redden by increasing blood flow

**SEDATIVE:** calming, soothing, tranquilizing

**SPLENIC:** treets the spleen

**STOMACHIC:** tones the stomach and increases appetite

**STYPTIC:** stops bleeding when applied to wound

**SUDORIFIC:** induces sweating

**TONIC:** strengthens the body and restores vitality

**VASODILATOR:** dilates and opens blood vessels

**VERMIFUGE:** destroys parasitic worms

**VULNERARY:** heals wounds

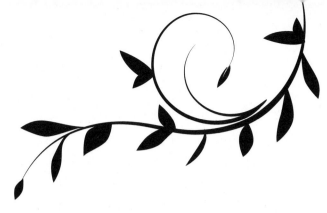

# REFERENCES

"A–Z Medicinal Herb Chart by Common Name." Annie's Remedy. Accessed April 12, 2018. http://www.anniesremedy.com/chart.php.

Alborzian, Yogi Cameron. *One Plan: A Week-by-Week Guide to Restoring Your Natural Health and Happiness*. New York: Harper One, 2014.

American College of Healthcare Sciences. "3 Common and Dangerous Essential Oil Mistakes | Achs.edu." Accredited Online Holistic Health College. Accessed April 30, 2018. http://info.achs.edu/blog /aromatherapy-essential-oil-dangers-and-safety.

"Aromatherapy & Essential Oils for Relaxation and Stress Relief." WebMD. Accessed February 22, 2018. https://www.webmd.com /balance/stress-management/aromatherapy-overview.

Bricklin, Mark, Cameron Stauth, Holly Clemson, Lloyd Rosenvold, and John Heinerman. *Rodale's Encyclopedia of Natural Home Remedies: Hundreds of Simple Healing Techniques for Everyday Illness and Emergencies*. Emmaus, PA: Rodale Press, 1982.

Chopra, Deepak. "Nutrition and Recipes Resources." The Chopra Center. May 12, 2016. Accessed September 1, 2016. https://chopra .com/nutrition-and-recipes.

"Complementary and Alternative Medicine (CAM)." WebMD. Accessed April 23, 2018. https://www.webmd.com/balance/guide /what-is-alternative-medicine.

"Deb Augur, Author at Herbs and Natural Remedies for Health." Herbs and Natural Remedies for Health. Accessed November 16, 2016. http://herbsandnaturalremedies.com/author/admin/.

Desy, Phylameana Lila. "Coping Tips for Anyone Suffering with Tinnitus." ThoughtCo. March 17, 2017. Accessed August 8, 2018. https://www.thoughtco.com/how-to-deal-with-tinnitus-1729532.

Dodt, Colleen K. *The Essential Oils Book: Creating Personal Blends for Mind & Body*. Pownal, VT: Storey, 1996.

"Essential Oils and Pregnancy: Pregnancy: First Trimester Community–Support Group." WebMD. Accessed February 28, 2018. https://forums.webmd.com/3/pregnancy-first-trimester-exchange /forum/19158.

Ferrell, Vance, and Harold M. Cherne. *Natural Remedies Encyclopedia: America's Master Book of House Remedies*. Altamont, TN: Harvestime, 2004.

Fite, Vannoy Gentles. *Essential Oils for Emotional Wellbeing: More than 400 Aromatherapy Recipes for Mind, Emotions & Spirit*. Woodbury, MN: Llewellyn, 2018.

Fite, Vannoy Gentles, Michele Gentles McDaniel, and Vannoy Lin Reynolds. *Essential Oils for Healing: Over 400 All-Natural Recipes for Everyday Ailments*. New York: St. Martin's, 2016.

Frawley, David. *Yoga and Ayurveda: Self-Healing and Self-Realization*. Delhi: Motilal Banarsidass, 2013.

———. *Ayurveda Healing: A Comprehensive Guide*. Delhi: Motilal Banarsidass, 1992.

Kalish, Nancy. "10 Best Healing Herbs." *Prevention*. November 31, 2011. Accessed August 8, 2016. https://www.prevention.com/life/ a20467532/best-healing-herbs-top-10/.

Keville, Kathi, and Mindy Green. *Aromatherapy: A Complete Guide to the Healing Art*. Vancouver, BC: Langara College, 2016.

Kowalchik, Claire, William H. Hylton, and Anna Carr. *Rodale's Illustrated Encyclopedia of Herbs*. Emmaus, PA: Rodale Press, 1998.

Lad, Vasant. *The Complete Book of Ayurvedic Home Remedies*. London: Piatkus, 2006.

"Mayo Clinic: The Integrative Guide to Good Health." BlogTalkRadio. August 08, 2017. Accessed September 16, 2017. http://www.blogtalkradio.com/feisty-side-of-fifty/2017/08/08/mayo-clinic-the-integrative-guide-to-good-health.

Parramore, Karin. *Aromatherapy with Essential Oil Diffusers: For Everyday Health & Wellness*. Toronto: Robert Rose, 2017.

Shealy, C. Norman. *Illustrated Encyclopedia of Healing Remedies*. New York: HarperCollins, 2002.

Sondhi, Amrita. *The Modern Ayurvedic Cookbook: Healthful, Healing Recipes for Life*. Vancouver, BC: Arsenal Pulp Press, 2014.

Spear, Heidi E. *The Everything Guide to Chakra Healing*. Avon, MA: Adams Media, 2011.

Worwood, Susan E., and Valerie Ann Worwood. *Essential Aromatherapy: A Pocket Guide to Essential Oils and Aromatherapy*. Novato, CA: New World Library, 2003.